The Guide to HEALTHY EATING

2nd Edition

David Brownstein, M.D. & Sheryl Shenefelt, C.N.

For further copies of *The Guide To Healthy Eating, 2nd Edition*

Order online: www.drbrownstein.com or www.sherylshenefelt.com

Call: **1-888-647-5616** or send a check or money order in the amount of: $23.00 ($18.00 plus $5.00 shipping and handling) or for Michigan residents $24.08 ($18.00 plus $5.00 shipping and handling, plus $1.08 sales tax) to:

> Healthy Living
> 964 Floyd Street
> Birmingham, Michigan 48009

Acknowledgements

David Brownstein, M.D.

I gratefully acknowledge the help I have received from my friends and colleagues in putting this book together. This book could not have been published without help from the editors— my wife Allison and my chief editor Janet Darnell.

I would also like to thank my patients. It is your search for safe and effective natural treatments that is the driving force behind holistic medicine. You have accompanied me down this path and I appreciate each and every one of you.

And, finally, I would like to thank my staff. From the bottom of my heart THANK YOU! Thank you for believing in me and believing in what we do. Without your help, this would not be possible.

Sheryl Shenefelt, CN

I am extremely grateful to all of the help and support I received from my family, friends, and clients in putting this book together and in my ongoing quest for nutrition information and optimal health. I am thankful to the relationship both as a friend and co-worker, to Dr. David Brownstein for the opportunity to write this book and the process of sharing insightful ideas, not to mention working with him and his patients.

I also appreciate the work of Lisa Capraro and Healthy Traditions Network (local chapter of the Weston A. Price Foundation) for inspiring and connecting me to all of the wonderful resources that initially guided me in my quest for real information and real food. Finally, to my three favorite people, my husband Bob, daughter Grace, and son Nicholas, for their patience and ongoing love and support.

How to Utilize this Book

➢ What should I eat?

➢ How do I cook healthy food?

➢ How do I shop for healthy food?

These are questions that we, as a doctor and a nutritionist, hear daily from our clients, patients, friends, and families. The first step to attaining a healthier lifestyle includes learning which foods to eat and which foods to avoid. Healthy food is not found in a box or a package. Healthy food is found in the form of whole food, not refined food. The information in this book can help you make better food choices to improve both your health and your family's health.

The goal of this book is to provide some basic insights and resources as well as to expose some misconceptions about nutrition and food. The Guide to Health Eating, 2nd Edition is simply that: A GUIDE! This book is filled with research, easy-to-follow steps for making the right food choices, healthy eating tips, grocery shopping tips and recipes to assist you in healthy eating.

It is organized in easy-to-read chapters based on nutrition topics such as protein, carbohydrates, fats, etc. Each chapter starts with a Frequently Asked Question (FAQ) section that will provide you with information on these topics. This is followed by the Simple Steps and Replacements that can help you implement healthy changes in your diet. You don't have to do everything at once. Use the book as a reference and pick one section to focus on, and then come back to the following section when you are ready to make the next transition. The final part of each chapter provides Meal Ideas intended to assist you in your selection of daily meals and snacks. Several recipes are suggested that exemplify what has been expressed in the chapters. The recipes are easy to follow. Try one at a time.

In this 2nd edition we have added two new chapters "Foods to Eat and Foods to Avoid" and " What to Buy at the Grocery Store" to help you make better choices while grocery shopping and even to offer our opinion on optimal brand selections. Also we have added a "Tips Section" to guide you on everything from organic and local buying, dining out and recipe conversion to food preparation, meal planning and cooking. We hope you can use the information and resources in this book to guide you on your quest for healthy eating!

A Word of Caution to the Reader

The information presented in this book is based on the training and professional experience of the authors. The advice in this book should not be undertaken without first consulting a physician. Proper laboratory and clinical monitoring is essential to achieving the goals of finding safe and effective natural treatments. This book was written for informational and educational purposes only. It is not intended to be used as medical advice.

Dedications

David Brownstein, M.D.

To the women of my life: Allison, Hailey and Jessica, with all my love.

And, to my patients. Thank you for being interested in what I am interested in.

Sheryl Shenefelt, CN

With love to my wonderful husband Bob and beautiful children Grace and Nicholas.

Contents

Preface
David Brownstein, M.D.

In medical school, I received no training on how to give my patients dietary advice. I was taught how to diagnose illnesses and how to prescribe and utilize drugs to treat these illnesses. There was little mention about dietary choices or the importance of diet in not only treating an illness, but in promoting health.

Eighteen years of medical practice has proven to me that prescription medications are not the most powerful drugs available to physicians and patients. The most powerful drugs are readily attainable every day, in fact, in most cases, at least three times a day. We access the most powerful drugs every time we eat. The content of our food is a primary factor in determining whether our health is good or bad. Simply stated, good food is fundamental to good health.

Eating the wrong food will lead to advanced signs of aging, as well as the onset and exacerbation of chronic illness. So where do people go for information on how to improve their diet? Many conventional organizations parrot the same advice – "Follow the food pyramid." Mainstream physicians, the American Diabetic Association, AMA, and most dieticians promote the Standard American Diet (SAD) as illustrated by the food pyramid. The SAD has been a disaster for our country. We face an epidemic of obesity, hypertension, cancer, heart disease, diabetes, fatigue, fibromyalgia and other illnesses that are caused, in part, by the SAD diet.

My experience as a holistic physician has clearly shown that better food choices lead to an enhanced immune system and an overall improvement in one's health.

Nutritional food contains vitamins, minerals, enzymes, and other healing agents for our bodies. Refined food, including refined sugar, salt, and grains, contains little or no healthful nutrients. The food industry has aggressively promoted the use of refined foods since they are inexpensive to manufacture and have a long shelf life.

Refined food not only provides no nutrients for the body, it actually depletes the body of its store of vitamins, minerals, and enzymes. A healthier approach is to use whole, unrefined food. Unrefined food actually contains healthy nutrients, which supply our bodies with the basic raw materials that promote healing.

One of the most repeated questions I get from my patients is, "What food should I eat?" This book provides you with a concise, easy-to-follow guide on how to implement a healthier lifestyle by improving your diet to include healthier food.

To All of Our Health!

Sheryl Shenefelt, CN

Most of my initial interest in nutrition came from reading magazine articles and trying new recipes. My knowledge was shaped by what I found in these magazines, what I saw on TV, or whatever the latest "fad" was. While in college, I was just like other girls, always trying to watch my weight, eating low-fat foods, and buying things in packages that the commercials or the ads on the boxes claimed were healthy for me. Soon my health began to deteriorate and I had low blood sugar and extreme fatigue. With the desire to take control of my health and well-being, I enrolled in massage therapy school where I learned more about how the body functions. I realized that food was important and that the information put out by the media just didn't make sense. I focused more on natural, organic, and whole foods. As I started to feel better and regain energy, it became clear to me that having and maintaining optimal health involved a shift in lifestyle priorities.

The Weston A. Price Foundation, specifically the Detroit Chapter called Healthy Traditions Network, had a big influence on my food choices. I discovered that food can and should taste good while also fueling the body. I was surprised (and glad!) to find out that fat is actually an important and necessary food for healthy bodily functions and not something to be avoided in the hope of losing weight. I learned that fat is not what makes people obese; it is the refined foods that are so prevalent nowadays, such as white flour, white sugar, and hydrogenated oils. These refined foods should be avoided. As Hippocrates, the father of medicine, said: "Foods must be in the condition in which they are found in nature, or at least in a condition as close as possible to that found in nature."

At the time, these concepts were not so clear to me because I was living in a busy society with so many confusing nutrition messages both from the media and from the huge corporations who profit from the foods we buy. With such a fast-paced world, it is no wonder that many people have turned to prepackaged, processed, convenience foods which are devoid of nutrients, and it is unfortunate that their health takes the toll. The primary goal of food manufacturers is not nutrition quality. Their goal is to have a long shelf life for their products and large profit margins.

From my experience as a nutritionist and also as a wife and mother desiring a healthy family, I recognize the importance of carefully selecting the type of food we eat, knowing where our food comes from, and buying foods in their most natural state from local farmers whenever possible. In my consultations and classes, clients are always confused about healthy food -- what to eat, what food to buy and where to buy it, and how to identify healthy food.

The media, in my opinion, is not a reliable source for accurate information about nutrition. This book will provide you with the basics of nutrition. It will help you make better food choices, and help you improve your family's health.

1

Carbohydrates

Carbohydrates

Frequently Asked Questions

What are carbohydrates?

Carbohydrates provide quick fuel for the body in the form of sugars and starches, as well as fiber. Carbohydrates are found mostly in plant foods such as fruits, vegetables, grains, and potatoes. Milk also contains some carbohydrates.

Carbohydrates come in two basic forms: simple and complex. Simple carbohydrates are very small molecules of sugar (usually one or two molecules of sugar, such as table sugar), whereas complex carbohydrates, such as starches, contain many hundreds to thousands of sugar units linked together.

What are some of the differences between simple and complex carbohydrates?

Simple carbohydrates (e.g., sucrose or table sugar, and fruit) are very sweet to the taste and are digested very quickly by the body. Complex carbohydrates are pleasant to the taste, but they are not as sweet as simple carbohydrates, and they take longer to digest. Examples of simple and complex carbohydrates are shown in Table 1.

Table 1: Simple and Complex Carbohydrates

Simple Carbohydrates	Complex Carbohydrates
Fructose - fruit, honey, high fructose corn syrup	**Fiber** - whole wheat breads, cereals, oats, legumes, psyllium, rice bran, barley
Glucose - dextrose, corn syrup	
Lactose - milk, dairy	**Starches** - flour, bread, rice, corn, oats, barley, potatoes, legumes, vegetables
Sucrose - table sugar, brown sugar	

Which carbohydrates should I avoid?

All carbohydrates are not created equal. Unrefined carbohydrates, with their full complement of minerals, vitamins, enzymes, and fiber can be a healthy food choice. Unrefined carbohydrates contain naturally occurring sugars found in many food products such as fruits and vegetables. Refined carbohydrates, on the other hand, contain little or no nutrients and are not healthy for the body. Avoid refined carbohydrates in the form of white sugar, soft drinks, and candies that give you plenty of calories but little or no nutrients.

A diet of excess refined carbohydrates (e.g., white sugar) can lead to many nutritional deficiencies and poor health including increasing the incidence of chronic illnesses such as obesity, cancer, heart disease, and arthritis. For more information on sugar, see Chapter 2, "Sweeteners".

How are carbohydrates refined?

The process of refining carbohydrates entails taking out all of the healthy nutrients (e.g., vitamins, minerals, enzymes) and leaving only the sugar molecules. The reason the food industry refines so many different products is to extend the shelf life. Once healthy nutrients are removed from the food, there is nothing in the food that can go rancid. Refined food can often sit on a shelf forever. Since there is no expiration date for a refined product, it is less expensive for a food manufacturing company to put it on the shelf as compared to a whole food (unrefined) product that has an expiration date.

How do you know if a product is refined?

Anything in a package that has no expiration date is refined. White flour, white sugar, high fructose corn syrup, white pasta, and white rice are examples of common refined carbohydrates. In order to eat food that is the most nutritious for your body, it is our recommendation that you eliminate, or at least reduce, the amount of refined carbohydrates in your diet.

What effect do carbohydrates have on blood sugar in the body?

Our bodies can turn simple or refined carbohydrates into glucose (sugar) very quickly. Eating too many refined carbohydrates can cause problems with blood sugar regulation. The refined sugars (candy and soft drinks) and refined grains (white flour and white rice) cause blood sugar levels to rise more quickly than a whole food (unrefined) product. Unrefined carbohydrates, such as whole grains, are broken down more slowly, allowing blood sugar to rise more gradually. Eating a diet that is high in foods that cause a rapid rise in blood sugar may increase a person's risk of developing health problems, such as hormonal imbalances and diabetes.

What is the glycemic index and how is it related to blood sugar?

The glycemic index (shown in Appendix A, page 225) was developed to measure how quickly carbohydrates enter into the bloodstream as glucose. In order to keep blood sugar from rising, we recommend that you eat foods with a low glycemic index (i.e., those with an index <50%). Another way to keep blood sugar from rising is to eat carbohydrates in balance with other whole foods that contain protein, fat, and other nutrients which help slow the entry of sugar into the body.

Which carbohydrates should I eat?

Carbohydrates, specifically complex carbohydrates, can be a healthy part of one's diet if they are eaten in their unrefined form. Unrefined, complex carbohydrates contain vitamins, minerals, enzymes, and fiber which not only aid the digestive process but also help to replenish the body's stores of vital nutrients. Items like whole grains and fresh vegetables which supply nutrients such as vitamins, minerals, and fiber should predominate in the diet over refined carbohydrates (sugars). Remember, refined carbohydrates supply no nutrients to the body and will deplete the body's own nutrient stores.

What are whole grains?

Whole grains are one type of complex carbohydrate. Whole grains contain vitamins, minerals, fiber, and other nutrients that work together to protect our health. Whole grains contain many nutrients, are especially high in B-vitamins, and contain a wide range of minerals. Whole grains contain all three parts of the grain (the bran, germ, and endosperm) and are slower to break down, making it easier for your body to regulate them. See Table 2 for a list of some whole grains.

Table 2: Whole Grains	
Amaranth	Oats
Barley	Quinoa
Brown rice	Rye
Buckwheat	Sorghum
Bulgur (cracked wheat)	Spelt
Kamut	Teff
Millet	Wild rice

One caveat about grains is that they can be hard on the digestive system. For the most efficient digestion and utilization of grains in the body, soak them overnight to predigest them. One way to soak them is to mix them in some water with yogurt or lemon juice. For examples of soaking, see Chapter 10, "Recipes".

An additional advantage of soaking grains is that it allows for the breakdown of the phytic acid in the grain, which research shows can block some mineral absorption.

On the other hand, refined white flour with the germ and bran removed has been stripped of most nutrients. Food companies will often add synthetic vitamins and minerals to their refined grains. Don't be fooled by the list of enriched items added back into a product; it is still inferior to the whole grain. As is the case with all refined products, the refining process is done in order to prolong the shelf life indefinitely and increase profit margins. Avoid products that do not have an expiration date. Remember, any product that can sit on the shelf forever without going rancid has no nutritional value to the body and should be avoided.

What about gluten containing grains?

Gluten is a protein found in many grain products (e.g., wheat, rye and barley). Gluten is a very difficult-to-digest protein and can wreak havoc on the system particularly for someone with a leaky gut, Celiac Disease or with gluten sensitivity. See Table 3 for a list of common gluten containing grains.

Table 3: Common Gluten Containing Grains

Barley	Semolina
Bulgur	Spelt
Couscous	Triticale
Durum	Rye
Einkorn	Wheat bran
Kamut	Wheat germ
Malt	Wheat starch

Gluten sensitivity is extremely common. The numbers of people suffering with this illness are staggering. There are estimates that nearly 1 in 133 Americans suffer from celiac disease (with perhaps one in six having gluten sensitivity).

For those that are sensitive to gluten, its ingestion can lead to the immune system attacking itself, and to the development of many serious illnesses including: autoimmune illnesses, cancer, chronic fatigue syndrome, and arthritis. For more information on gluten, please refer to the authors' book *The Guide to a Gluten-Free Diet.*

What are the healthiest vegetables to include in the diet?

Eating a rainbow of colored vegetables (i.e., yellows, reds, purples, blues, and greens) is important to help maintain an optimal immune system. Variety is the important thing to get all of the beneficial nutrients. Some of the nutrients include: flavanoids (antioxidants), carotenes, fiber, and phytonutrients. Green is one of the most important colors to include in the diet. Green leafy vegetables like spinach, kale, chard, etc. are some of the most nutrient rich carbohydrates. The darker the leaves, the more nutrients the vegetable has.

Simple Diet Suggestions and Replacements

It is important to begin reading labels on packages – see shopping tips in Chapter 9, "What to Buy at the Grocery Store". Look for and avoid processed, refined carbohydrates (such as white flour, white sugar, white pasta, and white rice) found in most cereals, cookies, cakes, muffins, frozen dinners, and other items.

Refined carbohydrates are often found in a box, bag, or package. Remember, if the package does not have an expiration date on it, you should probably steer clear of it.

Suggestion #1: Avoid white flour breads.

Replacement: Choose whole grain breads such as sourdough, sprouted, or 100% whole wheat without additives or hydrogenated oils. For more on hydrogenated oils, see Chapter 3, "Fats and Oils".

Suggestion #2: Avoid white flour and sugar-laced crackers, snacks, and cookies.

Replacement: Choose whole grain crackers, snacks, and cookies without hydrogenated oils. If sweetened, look for those with natural sweeteners.

White flour-filled breads, crackers, pastas, cookies, cakes, and similar items are all highly refined foods. They are often full of extra sugars, additives, and even toxic hydrogenated oils. White flour has been refined and bleached for extra softness and whiteness. The refining process leaves only the endosperm part of the grain and removes the bran, germ, and husk.

Whole grains, on the other hand, retain nutrients found in the original grain because they are milled in their entirety and not refined. Items such as iron, niacin, thiamin, riboflavin, folate, B6, magnesium, zinc, and fiber can often be found in whole grains still intact. Even with nutrients artificially added, white flour foods are still a poor nutritional choice.

Suggestion #3: Avoid boxed cereals and pancake mixes.

Replacement: Make oatmeal or homemade pancakes/waffles with whole grains.

Boxed cereals and pancake mixes are extremely refined foods and often full of unnecessary sugars, additives, and flavorings. Many breakfast cereals are also very highly fortified foods, full of hard to digest synthetic vitamins and minerals added during processing that may not even have been present in the original product. In addition, the processing of cereals (including those found at health food stores) often involves high heat and high temperatures that can deplete or destroy nutrients.

Suggestion #4: Avoid canned fruits and vegetables.

Replacement: Choose fresh (or frozen) fruits and vegetables, especially lots of leafy greens and a variety of colors. Choose organic or local whenever possible. For more information on the benefits of eating organic and local, see Tips Section II, page 199.

Canned fruits and vegetables often have unnecessary syrups, salts, and other additives to make them last for long periods of time on the shelf. Fresh fruits and vegetables offer greater nutrient availability (e.g., antioxidant flavonoids), especially if organic is selected. Frozen is always a great alternative when fresh is unavailable, and frozen fruits and vegetables will still be more nutritious than canned.

Meal Ideas

The following ideas and recipes will show you how to utilize some healthier, unrefined carbohydrates in your eating plan. Grains, beans, and vegetables can add variation to your diet and are also healthy additions to meals.

Breakfast:
- ✓ whole grain waffles or pancakes
- ✓ whole grain bread and free-range, organic eggs for French toast
- ✓ whole grain muffins topped with butter
- ✓ oatmeal, barley, or quinoa cereal served with butter or coconut oil (Great with some kefir or yogurt on the side!)

Recipes:
- ✓ Carrot Spice Muffins, page 152
- ✓ Cinnamon Waffles, page 153
- ✓ French Toast, page 157

Lunch:
- ✓ bean and/or vegetable soups or stews
- ✓ salads or soups with green leafy vegetables and/or quinoa
- ✓ frittatas or casseroles full of fresh colorful vegetables
- ✓ fresh salad with various chopped vegetables, topped with nuts and homemade dressing
- ✓ tortillas with vegetables, beans, cheese, or hummus

Recipes:

- ✓ Chicken-Honey Mustard Salad, page 161
- ✓ Coconut Balsamic Salad, page 162
- ✓ Creamy Vegetable Bean Soup, page 163
- ✓ Lentil Sweet Potato Soup, page 164
- ✓ Mini Muffin Pizzas, page 164

Snacks:

- ✓ salsas or bean dips with vegetables or whole grain crackers
- ✓ raw cheese and nuts or whole grain crackers
- ✓ fresh chopped vegetables or fruit
- ✓ lettuce wraps with hummus

Recipes:

- ✓ Hummus Dip, page 185
- ✓ Pineapple Chipotle Salsa, page 186
- ✓ Simply Salsa, page 187

Dinner:

- ✓ vegetable sides with your meals (lots of leafy greens)
- ✓ grains mixed in squash or vegetable dishes
- ✓ rice or quinoa instead of potatoes for a side dish
- ✓ vegetable and rice stir fry
- ✓ fresh salad with colored peppers and other vegetables

Recipes:

- ✓ Coconut Green Beans, page 181
- ✓ Ginger Quinoa Squash, page 182
- ✓ Lemon Tahini Kale, page 183
- ✓ Sloppy Lentils, page 170
- ✓ Vegetable Rice Stir Fry, page 173

2

Sweeteners

Sweeteners

Frequently Asked Questions

How common are sweeteners in the diet?

Who *doesn't* have a sweet tooth? Sweetening food to make it more palatable has been done since the beginning of time. However, using too much of a good thing or substituting a fake sweetener for a natural sweetener can cause health problems. Americans, in particular, have a huge sweet tooth. We consume over 33% of the world's sugar, which amounts to over 10 million tons annually.[1] It is no wonder that America is suffering from an obesity problem.

This chapter will teach you why it is important to choose natural sweeteners while avoiding the refined and artificial ones. See the recipes in Chapter 10 for guidance on how to get started using natural sweeteners in your cooking.

What is the most common sweetener used?

The sugar most used today, commonly available at grocery stores, is white refined sugar. The refining process of sugar involves stripping the vitamins, minerals, and nutrients from it. The main reason food manufacturers refine sugar is to extend its shelf life. Refined sugar, devoid of all of its healthy nutrients (vitamins, minerals, and enzymes) can literally stay on the shelf forever, which increases the profit margin.

What are examples of refined sugar?

Sugar can either be refined or unrefined. Refined sugar, the most common sugar in use in the United States, is found in grocery stores as white sugar (e.g., table sugar). Table 4 lists some of the sources of refined sugar generally in use today. Agave, although used to be considered a good alternate sweetener, has since been found to not be as healthy as once thought as it is highly processed as well as high in fructose that contributes to fat storage. We suggest you avoid it.

Table 4: Refined Sugars
Agave
Brown Sugar
High Fructose Corn Syrup
Powdered Sugar
Turbinado Sugar
White Sugar

What effect does refined sugar have on the body?

Refined sugar depresses the immune system and can actually make the body deficient of vitamins and minerals. This occurs because the refining process of sugar (similar to the refining process for all foods) strips the healthy items--vitamins, minerals, and enzymes--from the plant product. In order to properly digest excess sugar, the body will be required to use its own store of nutrients, particularly many B vitamins. In addition, refined forms of sugar provide the body with the rush of the sugary taste and the quick elevation of blood sugar levels without the balancing effect of the healthful nutrients. The consumption of large amounts of refined sugar causes blood glucose (sugar) swings in the body and may lead to the development of many chronic illnesses including diabetes, arthritis, and cancer, as well as many other serious health conditions, as seen in Table 5.

Table 5: Problems Associated with Refined Sugar

Arthritis	Heart Disease
Asthma	Hyperactivity
Cancer	Infections
Candida	Immune System Illnesses
Dental Decay	Kidney Disease
Depression	Liver Disease
Diabetes	Obesity
Headaches	Osteoporosis

Are artificial sugar substitutes a healthy alternative to refined sugar?

No, these products are often toxic to the body and need to be avoided. Sugar substitutes are recommended by many physicians and health agencies, including the American Diabetic Association, as a way to lose weight. The United States uses more artificial sweeteners than any other country. Presently, the United States is the most obese country. The research shows that the use of artificial sweeteners does not prevent obesity.

Sugar substitutes are known as aspartame (AminoSweet®, NutraSweet®, as well as Equal®, Spoonful®, and Equal-Measure®), saccharin (Sweet'N Low®), and sucralose (Splenda®).

The most common artificial sweetener used is aspartame. The United States consumes over 80% of the world's supply of aspartame. It is added to more than 6,000 foods and many pharmaceuticals, including many children's liquid medications.

Our experience has shown that consuming large amounts of aspartame may actually cause many health problems, including obesity. We have found that it is very difficult for people to lose weight if they are consuming large amounts of aspartame. In addition, there are many neurological disorders and immune system disorders exacerbated by aspartame. Aspartame should not be used in any amount and needs to be avoided.

Sucralose is a newer sweetener marketed as Splenda®. However, sucralose, which has two chlorine molecules per molecule of sucralose, can lead to thyroid and other hormonal problems. Sucralose should be avoided.

Should I avoid all sweeteners?

Not necessarily. The sweetening of food, whether for desserts or meals, is important in that it serves the purpose of making food a pleasurable experience. Many people are unaware that there are unrefined and natural sweeteners available that taste good and yet also contain helpful vitamins or minerals. We suggest you eat natural sweeteners in moderation along with a meal or snack that also includes good quality fat or protein.

What are natural sweetener alternatives to refined sugar?

There are a variety of sources of natural sweeteners that can enhance the taste of food while also providing some essential vitamins and minerals. Unrefined and natural sweeteners should be used in moderation in one's diet, optimally accompanied by some good proteins or fats to prevent a spike and crash in blood sugar. Table 6 gives examples of sweeteners that could be used in your recipes for a more natural alternative to white sugar in your diet.

Table 6: Natural Sweeteners

Fruit (bananas, strawberries, blueberries, etc)
Coconut Palm Sugar
Honey (raw)
Maple sugar
Maple syrup
Molasses
Rapadura
Stevia
Sucanat
Xylitol

How do the various natural sweeteners differ?

Coconut Palm Sugar

Coconut palm sugar is ideally the type made by evaporating the sap from the coconut blossoms into crystals. It is not high in fructose and has a somewhat low glycemic index at just 35 for about two tablespoons. (See Appendix A for more on glycemic index). It is also a source of minerals, vitamin C, B vitamins, and some amino acids.

Honey

Raw honey is often thought to be one of the most nutritious sweeteners due to its high enzyme and nutrient content. Raw honey has trace amounts of potassium, calcium, and phosphorus and is well known for its healing antiseptic, antibacterial, and antifungal properties.

Maple Sugar

Maple sugar is dehydrated maple syrup. It seems to have arisen from the traditions of the Native American Indians. Maple sugar contains the nutrients potassium, calcium, as well as trace minerals.

Maple Syrup

Maple syrup is a good source of manganese, zinc, and other nutrients. Grade B syrup is less refined than the grade A, so it holds more of the nutrients and it also has a stronger taste.

Molasses

Blackstrap molasses is the dark liquid byproduct of the process of refining sugar cane into table sugar. Blackstrap molasses is a wonderful source of iron, as well as calcium, copper, potassium, and magnesium that add to its nutritious value.

Rapadura

Rapadura is an unrefined and unbleached whole cane sugar. It is not separated from the molasses stream during processing, and retains some nutrient value such as potassium, calcium, and magnesium. It can be used to replace both white and brown sugar.

Stevia

Stevia is an herb that can be used as a powder extract or a liquid concentrate for varying levels of sweetness. Stevia may take a little getting used to, because sometimes it will have a slight aftertaste. Notably, Stevia does not seem to trigger a rise in blood sugar and has become a popular alternative to artificial sweeteners.

Sucanat

Sucanat is extracted from sugar cane by a squeezing process. The juice that is crystallized does not have the molasses removed and thus retains nutrient value. It is a great replacement for both white and brown sugars, and is especially good for baking.

Xylitol

This sweetener is just as sweet as table sugar, but with about one-third the calories. As a low-glycemic sweetener, it is safe for diabetics and hypoglycemics. Xylitol has also been shown to decrease the incidence of tooth decay.

How can I use natural sweeteners instead of refined sugar in my recipes?

The following table and the dessert recipes in this book will assist you in making easy, good-tasting items that are much healthier when made with natural sweeteners as compared to refined sugar and artificial substitutes.

Table 7: Conversion for 1 cup of White Sugar

Coconut Palm Sugar	1 for 1 replacement white or brown sugar
Honey (raw)	⅔ cup and reduce any liquids in recipe by ¼ cup
Maple Sugar	¾ cup
Maple Syrup	¾ cup and reduce any liquids in recipe by 3 tablespoons
Molasses (Blackstrap)	⅔ cup and reduce liquids in recipe by 5 tablespoons
Rapadura	1 for 1 replacement white or brown sugar
Stevia	⅛- ¼ teaspoon
Sucanat	1 for 1 replacement white or brown sugar
Xylitol	1 for 1 replacement
General rules: If substituting a liquid form of sweetener for a dry form of sweetener then either decrease the liquids in the recipe by ¼ cup for every cup of sweetener that you are using, or add an extra ¼ cup of flour.	

Simple Diet Suggestions and Replacements

Refined sugar has no place in a healthy diet. It leads to many health problems including cancer and degenerative diseases. Any sweetener should be used in moderation and, when sweetening a product, use a natural sweetener.

Suggestion #1: Avoid white sugar, high fructose corn syrup, candy bars, and other refined sugar items in many common packaged foods.

Replacement: Make your own desserts or buy products made with natural sweeteners.

Many packaged store-bought cakes, cookies, candies, and desserts are full of refined sugar or high fructose corn syrup. In order to process refined sugar, our bodies have to use up their store of vitamins and minerals to properly digest it. The intake of large amounts of refined sugar will lead to depletion of vitamins and minerals and, eventually, the development and acceleration of chronic illness.

By making your own desserts or buying desserts with natural sweeteners, you can still enjoy sweetness while benefiting from the added nutrient value found in natural sweeteners.

Suggestion #2: Avoid soft drinks and juice concentrates full of sugars and additives.

Replacement: Drink more water to quench thirst and try adding a bit of lemon, lime, or orange. Or you could squeeze your own fresh juices. Drink juices diluted with water for less concentrated sugar intake (this is especially important for children).

Soft drinks are one of the leading sources of unnecessary refined sugars in the diet, especially in children. Soft drinks have absolutely no nutritional value and are full of additives, extra sugars, and extra calories. Most people can fill up on soft drinks and have little appetite for the real food their body needs. Additionally, concentrated fruit juices are a source of excess sugar without the balancing effects of the fiber that occurs in the natural fruit.

Suggestion #3: Avoid artificial sweeteners such as aspartame (e.g., Equal®, NutraSweet®, AminoSweet®) and sucralose (e.g., Splenda®) that are toxic to the body.

Replacement: Use natural sweeteners or fruit.

Sugar substitutes are extremely toxic and often detrimental to one's health. Sugar substitutes do not promote weight loss, and many studies seem to indicate that individuals that use these products often gain more weight while using them. Natural sweeteners and fruit can be used safely as they do not have harmful chemicals or toxins that can cause imbalance in the body.

Meal Ideas

There are many natural sweeteners that can provide numerous healthy vitamins and minerals to our diet. The meal ideas below will help you integrate these items into your diet to replace white sugar and artificial sweeteners. It is important to remember that even natural sweeteners should be used in moderation and should be eaten along with high quality fats and proteins rather than by themselves.

Breakfast:
- ✓ organic maple syrup on pancakes, waffles, or French toast
- ✓ raw honey and cinnamon with oatmeal
- ✓ maple syrup and vanilla in yogurt or kefir
- ✓ natural sweeteners or fresh fruit in smoothies
- ✓ fresh fruit

Recipes:
- ✓ Cinnamon Waffles, page 153
- ✓ French Toast, page 157
- ✓ Healthy Smoothie, page 158
- ✓ Yogurt-Seed Surprise, page 158

Lunch:
- ✓ fresh fruit on sandwiches
- ✓ dried or fresh fruit in salads
- ✓ natural sweeteners for dressings

Recipes:

- ✓ Almond Butter Sandwich, page 159
- ✓ Coconut Balsamic Salad, page 162

Snacks:

- ✓ dried fruit in trail mixes
- ✓ natural sweeteners in salsas, dips, and spreads

Recipes:

- ✓ Almighty Almonds Trail Mix, page 188
- ✓ Nuts for Chocolate Trail Mix, page 188
- ✓ Pecan Surprise Trail Mix, page 188
- ✓ Pineapple Chipotle Salsa, page 186

Dinner:

- ✓ raw honey over sweet potatoes or squash
- ✓ natural sweeteners in sauces and stews
- ✓ blackstrap molasses for basting to add a rich color and taste

Recipes:

- ✓ Ginger Quinoa Squash, page 182
- ✓ Sweet Potato Fries, page 183

Dessert:

Replace the white sugar in your recipes with natural sweeteners using the previously mentioned conversion chart on page 43. For chocolate lovers, try cocoa or some chocolate extract to give that chocolate flavor—or try good quality organic chocolate!

Ideas:

- ✓ fresh fruit (try topped with organic cream)
- ✓ homemade fruit pies and cobblers
- ✓ homemade cakes and pudding
- ✓ macaroons
- ✓ custard

Recipes:

- ✓ Almond Butter-Coconut Crust, page 174
- ✓ Apple Bars, page 175
- ✓ Applesauce Cake, page 176
- ✓ Baked Custard, page 177
- ✓ Chocolate Brownie Cake, page 178
- ✓ Chocolate-Fudgy Frosting, page 178
- ✓ Cocoa-nut Milk Pudding, page 179
- ✓ Cocoa-nut Milk Pudding Bars, page 179
- ✓ Nutty Fruit Cobbler, page 180

---

[1] WHO

3

Fats and Oils

Fats and Oils

Frequently Asked Questions

What is fat?

Food consists of three major macronutrients: carbohydrates, protein, and fat. Fat contains more energy than either protein or carbohydrates. Fat is essential for forming cell membranes and for hormone production. Inadequate fat intake can lead to vitamin deficiency since fat acts as a carrier for fat-soluble vitamins, including Vitamins A, D, E, and K. Fat is found in both animal and vegetable products, adds flavor to food, and satisfies hunger as well. This chapter will review why <u>good fats</u> are essential to maintaining health.

Should I eat a low-fat diet?

The American public has been told by organizations such as The American Medical Association, The American Cancer Society, dieticians, their own physicians, and our government that we must eat low-fat foods in order to be healthy. However, numerous imbalances and vitamin deficiencies, including Vitamins A, D, E, and K, are apparent in low-fat diets. The low-fat idea is emphasized in the food pyramid that is so well known. Even with the recent changes to the food pyramid, little emphasis is on fat in the diet; and the most emphasis is on grains. And, there is no information promoted about why it is important to ingest adequate amounts of healthy fats.

Is the food pyramid a reliable guide to a healthy diet?

The food pyramid reflects the standard American diet. In the last 20 years, fat consumption has decreased 11% in this country. What has been the result of 20 years of following a diet low in fat and high in carbohydrates? It has made Americans the most obese people on this planet. In fact, during the last 20 years, while fat intake has decreased, obesity has increased 32%![1]

The standard American diet is a major cause of the tremendous growth of degenerative disorders seen in this country including autoimmune disorders, cancer, arthritis, coronary artery disease, and many others. Also, this diet promotes an imbalanced hormonal system. In order to promote health, we must understand the important role food has in providing fuel and nutrients for our bodies. In turn, we will be able to understand how to use food, including healthy fats, to provide our bodies with essential nutrients to promote true healing.

Why do I need fat in my diet?

Many people have a fear that fats lead to weight gain and so they avoid cooking or baking with them. However, adequate intake of good fats from whole foods gives satiety, which makes us less likely to overeat. Every cell membrane in the body contains fat, and all steroid hormones are produced from the fat-like substance, cholesterol. Cholesterol is an important molecule for the body. Without adequate amounts of cholesterol, hormone production will not occur and the immune system will not function optimally. In addition, protein cannot be adequately utilized without proper amounts of fat in the diet. Because fat is so important to our overall health, ingesting the wrong types of fat may promote a poor immune system, poor healing capacity, and a malfunctioning hormonal system.

What are good and bad fats?

Good fats are fats that the body can use to maintain structure and produce energy. Good fats come in many different forms. They are naturally occurring in food. Our bodies can use good fats to maintain healthy immune and hormonal systems.

Good fats are those that have not been hydrogenated and can be in the form of saturated, monounsaturated, or polyunsaturated.

Bad fats not only provide no nutrition to the body, but also cause the immune system to malfunction and lead to a variety of illnesses from obesity to cancer and autoimmune problems. Examples of bad fats are shown in Table 8.

Table 8: Bad Fats

- Partially Hydrogenated Vegetable Oils
- Processed Vegetable Oils (e.g., soy, canola, corn, and cottonseed)
- Trans Fats

What are saturated fats and should I avoid them?

Saturated fats have received a bad rap from physicians and dieticians as well as the media. Saturated fats have no double bonds and have all the hydrogen atoms that they can hold onto, making these fats very stable. Stable fats can withstand cooking at higher heat without producing tissue damaging free radicals. Saturated fats are solid or firm at room temperature and come mainly from animal sources such as meat and dairy products.

Optimal health is not possible without adequate amounts of saturated fats in our bodies. Saturated fats give our cells the strength to maintain structure and, since they predominate in our brains, they are especially crucial for a baby's brain development.

What are sources of saturated fats?

Different sources of saturated fats are listed in Table 9. Saturated fats, from the right sources, can provide important nutrition for the body.

Table 9: Healthy Foods That Contain Significant Amounts of Saturated Fats
Coconut Oil
Cultured Dairy (i.e. yogurt, kefir)
Organic Butter
Organic, Free-Range Red Meat
Palm Oil

What are monounsaturated fats?

Monounsaturated fats are liquid at room temperature and are known for being particularly high in the antioxidant Vitamin E. Monounsaturated fats are missing a hydrogen pair giving them one double bond in their chemical structure. The more double bonds a fat has, the less stable it is for cooking and high heat temperatures. Since monounsaturated fats are not as stable for cooking, they are best used in spreads and dressings or occasional lower heat cooking.

What are sources of monounsaturated fats?

The most common form of a monounsaturated fat is called oleic acid and is found in the items listed below in Table 10.

Table 10: Sources of Monounsaturated Fat

Avocado	Macadamias
Almonds	Olive Oil
Canola Oil	Peanuts
Cashews	Pecans
Hazelnuts	Pistachios

What is wrong with hydrogenated oils?

Partially hydrogenated vegetable oils are highly refined oils and are found in most packaged foods. Hydrogenation is a process used to convert liquid vegetable oils to solid or semi-solid fats, such as margarine. The process artificially adds hydrogen to their double bonds, making their chemical structure more stable.

The only benefits to hydrogenation are for the manufacturers. These fats are inexpensive to produce, and they also have an extremely long shelf life, making them ideal for commercially packaged foods. The downside for consumers is the dangerous trans fats that are formed with hydrogenation. The ingestion of partially hydrogenated vegetable oils and the trans fats that are formed with this process has been linked to increases in cancer, heart disease, and many other chronic degenerative disorders.

What is wrong with trans fats?

Trans fats, formed during hydrogenation, are actually toxic substances for our cell membranes. When our cells contain an overabundance of trans fats, the cells become leaky and distorted. This can promote vitamin and mineral deficiencies.

Trans fats are the most common fats found in many processed foods, including cookies, cakes, crackers, etc. Trans fats are not only toxic substances, they also block the proper absorption of good fats and need to be avoided, particularly by children and by those with a chronic illness.

What are polyunsaturated fats?

Polyunsaturated fats are missing two or more hydrogen pairs, or have two or more double bonds in their chemical structure (multiple double bonds make them even less stable than monounsaturated fats). Oils high in these fats are also liquid or soft at room temperature. Examples of oils high in polyunsaturated fatty acids are corn, safflower, soybean, and sunflower. Polyunsaturated oils are the least stable of all the fats and cannot withstand a lot of high heat processing or cooking because free radicals are easily formed. Free radicals are compounds that damage the cells of the body and contribute to diseases such as cancer, autoimmune disorders, obesity, and heart disease.

The most common forms of polyunsaturated fats in our diet are the Omega-6 (linoleic) and the Omega-3 (linolenic) fatty acids. Examples of both polyunsaturated fatty acids are shown in Table 11 below.

Table 11: Sources of Polyunsaturated Oils

Omega-3 Fatty Acids	Omega-6 Fatty Acids
Cold Water Fish Oils	Borage
(mackerel, salmon, albacore	Black Currant
tuna, sardines, lake trout)	Canola
Flax Seeds	Corn
Flaxseed Oil	Cottonseed
Pumpkin Seeds	Primrose
Walnuts	Safflower
	Soybean
	Sunflower

What is wrong with processed polyunsaturated (i.e., vegetable) oils such as soy, corn, canola, cottonseed, etc?

Processed vegetable oils (i.e., refined oils) are extremely abundant in today's diets and are the most common oils found at grocery stores. These oils are overused due to misinformation of their health qualities by the food industry as well as many health care providers. They contain high amounts of Omega-6 without the balancing effects of Omega-3, and have been shown to depress the immune system over time. In addition, many of these oils (soybean, canola, corn, and cottonseed) contain harmful free radicals due to the high heat and pressures of the refining process.

What are essential fatty acids?

The polyunsaturated forms called Omega-3 and Omega-6 oils are termed "Essential Fatty Acids". They are essential because the body cannot manufacture them. Life itself is not possible without adequate amounts of essential fatty acids.

Omega-6 and especially Omega-3 oils are very sensitive to heat and to modern food processing. Hydrogenation or high heat processing of these oils not only removes all of the nutrients from them, but also makes the oils toxic to our bodies by forming dangerous trans fats or free radicals that damage our cells. Also, essential fatty acids are not recommended for cooking due to their instability and sensitivity to heat. Omega-3 oils should never be heated and should only be added after cooking has been completed.

Do I need more Omega 3's in my diet?

Yes, the typical American diet consists of too many poor quality (i.e., refined or hydrogenated) Omega-6's. An unhealthy balance of Omega-6 oils is prevalent in common supermarket foods such as non-organic eggs, fish, and meat, as well as vegetable oils. It is important to have a properly balanced intake of healthy essential fats including both Omega-6 and Omega-3 fats.

Research has shown that an approximate ratio of 4:1 of healthy Omega-6:Omega-3 fat provides the body with a proper balance of essential fatty acids.

How can I use various fats and oils in cooking or as supplements?

It is important to be aware of the proper uses for good fats in order to get the most nutrients available and to avoid harmful substances (i.e. trans fats). The proper use of fats and oils depends on the chemical stability of the products, which is determined by the amounts of saturated, monounsaturated, and polyunsaturated fats within them. See Tables 12 and 13 for a summary of good fats and their appropriate uses as supplements and for cooking.

Table 12: Healthy Supplemental Oils:

Cod Liver Oil (never heat)	supplement for Vitamins A and D source of long chain essential fatty acids called EPA and DHA
Flaxseed Oil (never heat)	to add the balance of Omega-3's in salad dressings, spreads, dips in smoothies
High Vitamin Butter Oil (never heat)	source Activator X – aids mineral utilization (synergistic with cod)

Table 13: Healthy Cooking Oils:

Butter – preferably from grass-fed cattle (saturated fat)	replaces margarine light sautéing baking over vegetables or as a spread
Coconut Oil (saturated fat)	over vegetables or as spread cooking or baking in smoothies over popcorn
Extra Virgin Olive Oil (monounsaturated fat)	light sautéing (not as stable as coconut oil) salad dressings or over vegetables in spreads and condiments
Ghee or Clarified Butter (saturated fat)	replacement for casein sensitive higher smoke point than butter baking, stir frying dipping sauces or condiments
Palm Oil (saturated fat)	replaces shortening baking french fries
Peanut and Sesame oils	occasional stir frying
Safflower and Sunflower Oils (high oleic, expeller pressed)	use in balance with Omega-3's high oleic types can withstand some low heating

How can I purchase healthy oils?

It is important to consume high quality oils that have not been processed with unnecessary high heat and pressures. Table 14 will guide you in purchasing healthy cooking oils.

Table 14: How to Purchase Healthy Oils

1. The container must be shielded from light, as light damages healthy oils. Any clear container where you can see the oil should be avoided.

2. There should be an expiration date on the container. Nutrients have a shelf life. If there are no nutrients in the oil, they can stay on the shelf forever.

3. There should be no high temperature processing or hydrogenation of the oils, as these processes destroy the valuable nutrients and create toxins. (Look for expeller or cold pressed oils found mostly at health food stores.)

Simple Diet Suggestions and Replacements

Suggestion #1: Avoid processed vegetable oils such as canola, soy, cottonseed, corn, etc.

Replacement: Use coconut oil, palm oil, and/or olive oil.

Coconut and palm oil contain medium-chain fatty acids that are an important source of fast energy for the body. In addition, these items have potent antibacterial, antiviral, and anti-yeast properties. These saturated fats have also been found useful in aiding in the detoxification of the body. Interestingly, coconut oil has been shown to stimulate the body's metabolism which may facilitate weight loss.

Unrefined olive oil (extra virgin) can be used for light cooking or in salad dressing and spreads. Olive oil is very high in oleic acid, the most common form of monounsaturated fat.

Suggestion #2: Avoid margarine and other hydrogenated oils.

Replacement: Use butter or coconut oil.

Organic butter is one of the healthiest whole foods. It contains fat-soluble vitamins, trace minerals, short and medium-chain fats as well as other key nutrients. One of the most interesting items in butter (from cows grazing on grass) is the "X Factor", as described by Dr. Weston Price, one of the pioneers of using natural foods. The "X Factor" refers to a substance that helps the body absorb and utilize minerals.

Margarine, on the other hand, contains neither vitamins nor minerals. Margarine contains many substances harmful to the body, including trans-fatty acids formed during hydrogenation. Margarine should be avoided at all costs.

Meal Ideas

The following are some variations for using good fats and oils in the appropriate ways for cooking and baking. Some of the recipes call for coconut milk. About 10 ounces of coconut milk contains 3.5 tablespoons of coconut oil.

Breakfast:
- ✓ eggs cooked in butter or coconut oil
- ✓ smoothies made with coconut milk
- ✓ yogurt topped with nuts, seeds, or fresh fruit
- ✓ oatmeal topped with butter and/or coconut oil

Recipes:
- ✓ Cinnamon Coconut Oil Spread, page 190
- ✓ Egg Sandwich, page 156
- ✓ Honey Coconut Butter Spread, page 190
- ✓ Strawberry Coconut Butter Spread, page 190
- ✓ Yogurt-Seed Surprise, page 158

Lunch:
- ✓ salad with a good homemade dressing
- ✓ butter on bread for sandwiches
- ✓ vegetables sautéed or baked in coconut oil or olive oil

Recipes:
- ✓ Chicken-Honey Mustard Salad, page 161
- ✓ Coconut Balsamic Salad, page 162

- ✓ Coconut Green Beans, page 181
- ✓ Sweet Potato Fries, page 183

Snacks:

- ✓ smoothies with added cod liver oil or flax oil
- ✓ vegetables and dips made with olive or flax oils

Recipes:

- ✓ Guacamole Dip, page 184
- ✓ Healthy Smoothie, page 158
- ✓ Hummus Dip, page 185

Dinner:

- ✓ entrees cooked with butter and/or coconut oil
- ✓ lightly sauté vegetables with olive oil
- ✓ vegetables and sides served with butter

Recipes:

- ✓ Cheese Quesadillas, page 159
- ✓ Ginger Quinoa Squash, page 182
- ✓ Lemon Tahini Kale, page 183
- ✓ Sweet Potato Fries, page 183
- ✓ Vegetable Rice Stir Fry, page 173

---

[1] Heini, Adriann, et al. Divergent Trends in Obesity and Fat Intake Patterns: The American Paradox. American Journal of Medicine. March, 1997. vol. 102:26.

4

Protein

Protein

Frequently Asked Questions

What are proteins?

Proteins are the building blocks of the body, made up of amino acid chains. They are elements of every cell and necessary for building and repairing tissues. Proteins are also required for healthy muscles, skin, organs, the nervous system, and proper enzyme function.   In addition, the immune system uses specialized proteins called antibodies to fight infections. Optimal health is not possible without adequate amounts of quality sources of protein. Our experience has clearly shown that a poor intake of protein will lead to a cascade of medical problems including an inadequately functioning immune system and hormonal imbalances.

What are sources of protein?

Protein is found in both animal and plant products. However, animal protein is the only source of complete amino acids. Complete amino acids contain all of the essential amino acids. Protein from plant products is an incomplete source of protein in that it lacks some of the essential amino acids. Examples of animal and plant foods that contain sources of protein are shown in Table 15.

Table 15: Sources of Protein

Animal	Plant Family
Cheese	Beans
Eggs	Cereal
Fish	Corn
Meat	Legumes
Milk	Rice
	Soy

How is protein utilized in the body?

Protein cannot be utilized in the body without adequate amounts of fat. Nature has recognized this fact and, frequently, protein and fat are found together in healthy foods. Minerals are also necessary to properly digest and utilize protein. A balanced diet, including all of the essential nutrients, provides the body with all of the proper raw materials it needs to function optimally.

Is soy a healthy source of protein in the diet?

Soy is often touted in the media as a good source of protein. This information could not be farther from the truth. Soy is presently the cheapest crop to grow in the United States and, because it is widely available, it is being promoted as a healthy food. Soy contains enzyme inhibitors that block the absorption of many minerals essential in our bodies including: calcium, magnesium, zinc, molybdenum, manganese, and iron. If that is not bad enough, large amounts of refined soy can also cause deficiencies of Vitamins B12, D, E, and K. Fermented forms of soy (e.g., miso, natto, and tempeh) are much healthier than the typical soy eaten in the United States (e.g., soy milk, cheese, yogurt, hot dogs, burgers, etc.). Soy should not be the major source of protein in your diet. In fact, it would be best to eliminate all refined soy products from your diet. For more about soy see the authors' book *The Soy Deception*, as well as www.thesoydeception.com.

Is red meat a healthy source of protein in the diet?

Red meat can be a good source of protein particularly if it is grass-fed red meat or wild game. The best source of red meat is organic, which is free of antibiotics as well as hormones. Often vilified in the press, red meat contains the full complement of amino acids. Red meat not only contains many easily absorbable minerals, it also contains saturated fats. Saturated fats are necessary for proper brain function (the major fat in the brain is saturated fat) and they also provide strength to our cell walls.

Good saturated fats are essential to life. (For more on saturated fats, see Chapter 3, "Fats and Oils".)

Red meat contains B vitamins such as B2, B6, and B12. B12 is not found readily available in the plant family and many vegetarians may become deficient in Vitamin B12. Vitamins C and E are also found in meat, in addition to many minerals such as magnesium, zinc, selenium, and iron. Interestingly, in grass-fed meat there are higher amounts of beneficial conjugated linoleic acid (CLA). CLA has been noted for its anti-carcinogenic and body fat reducing effects.

Is poultry a healthy source of protein in the diet?

Poultry such as chicken and turkey can be a healthy source of protein if it is from organic, free-ranging animals able to access their natural diet. Another important factor to look for is poultry raised by farmers who do not use feed treated with pesticides and do not treat their stock with antibiotics or hormones. Poultry from a clean, healthy source is full of all of the essential amino acids and often noted for high tryptophan content. Poultry also provides phosphorus, selenium, niacin, and Vitamin B6.

Are eggs a healthy source of protein in the diet?

Eggs are the perfect food. Eggs contain the complete complement of amino acids, and also contain large amounts of the essential nutrients, choline and lutein. Organic, free-range eggs are a fantastic source of an ideal balance of Omega-3 and Omega-6 fats. Free-range eggs have a much better fatty acid profile than conventional chicken eggs. We recommend that you use only free-range, organic eggs in your diet.

Are beans and lentils a healthy source of protein in the diet?

Beans and lentils, although not complete proteins, can still be great sources of protein in the diet. Incomplete proteins are missing some of the essential amino acids, and yet can be combined with other incomplete proteins, such as grains, or with complete proteins, such as dairy, which also aid in their proper digestion. Some familiar combinations include rice and beans, trail mixes, and nut butters on toast.

Beans and lentils should be cleaned, rinsed, and soaked prior to cooking to loosen skins, ease in digestion, and also minimize cooking time and gassiness produced. Beans are inexpensive and extremely versatile, while also providing nutrients such as iron, zinc, potassium, magnesium, manganese, phosphorus, and thiamin.

Is fish a healthy source of protein?

Fish is very high in protein as well as a good source of many vitamins and minerals. Of specific importance is that fish contains Omega-3 fatty acids known for benefiting many areas of the body including the heart, brain, eyes, and joints. One caveat about eating fish is that the waters they swim in may contain pollution which can end up in the fish. Two of the most common pollutants include PCBs and mercury, which can both build up in the body over time. It is important to avoid fish with high levels of these toxic elements. The people that are the most sensitive to these toxins are young children and pregnant women. Wild-raised fish is the optimal choice for all of the wonderful health properties it holds. Many farm-raised fish not only have toxic items such as dyes and PCBs from the feed they are given, but also have an altered fatty acid profile as compared to wild fish.

Is dairy a healthy source of protein in the diet?

Commercial dairy products come from animals kept in confinement, fed hormones to fatten them, and given antibiotics to keep them alive. These are not healthy sources of protein. If dairy is desired in the diet, it is important to get organic forms of dairy (e.g., organic yogurt, kefir, and some raw cheeses) from animals not raised in confinement and that have access to their natural diet – grass.

Pasteurized milk (even organic) is not an optimal source of protein due to the alteration by both the homogenization and the pasteurization processes. Pasteurization denatures proteins, destroys enzymes and beneficial flora, as well as destroying nutrients such as Vitamin B6, B12, and C. The pasteurization process results in an altered structure of milk proteins that may be responsible for many of the milk allergies seen today. For those desiring to go dairy-free or required to go on a dairy-free diet, please see the authors' book *The Guide to a Dairy-Free Diet*.

Simple Diet Suggestions and Replacements

It is important to get protein in the diet, but it is especially important to get good quality, "clean" protein. Meats, for example, should be from animals not given antibiotics and hormones. Eggs should be from chickens ranging outside. Beans, nuts, and seeds should be organic (or at least raw, in the case of nuts).

Suggestion #1: Avoid commercially raised and/or grain-fed red meats.
Replacement: Organic and preferably grass-fed meats.

Suggestion #2: Avoid commercially raised chicken and turkey full of antibiotics, hormones, and growth stimulants.
Replacement: Organic and free-range chickens and turkeys not raised with antibiotics or hormones.

Commercially raised animals (the most common meat found in grocery stores and restaurants) are often raised in confinement without ever even seeing the light of day. They are given antibiotics for all of the diseases that arise due to their miserable living conditions. Moreover, synthetic growth hormones and stimulants are given in order to fatten these animals for slaughter and increase the profit margin.

Suggestion #3: Avoid commercially raised eggs found at most supermarkets.

Replacement: Buy organic, free-range eggs.

As mentioned in Chapter 3, it is important to have a balance of both Omega-6 and Omega-3 essential fatty acids in the diet. Commercially raised eggs, however, contain an excessive amount of Omega-6 with a ratio of about 20:1 with the Omega-3 fatty acids. By contrast, organic, free-range eggs have a ratio of approximately 2:1 Omega-6 to Omega-3 fatty acids and are, by far, the healthier choice in the diet.

Suggestion #4: Avoid processed meats such as bacon, sausage, and delicatessen meats full of nitrites and nitrates that are known carcinogens.

Replacement: Buy nitrite and nitrate-free meats from markets you trust.

Where can I buy good quality meats and fish?

Resources Online to Support Local Farmers

Local Harvest has a website that allows you to find all the farmers' markets, family farms, locally-grown produce, and grass-fed meats, along with other sources of sustainable food in your area. To find your area map, visit www.localharvest.org.

Eat Well Guide is a website that aids people in finding local producers, stores, and restaurants offering meat that is certified organic, raised without antibiotics or growth promoters, or raised in other sustainable methods. Visit www.eatwellguide.org.

Food Routes is a website promoting local food. An interactive map helps you connect to local farmers, Community Supported Agriculture, and farmers' markets in your area. Visit www.foodroutes.org.

Farmers' Markets are places to connect with local farmers that may provide some organic and pasture-raised products. Search for farmers' markets near you online at www.ams.usda.gov/farmersmarkets/map.htm.

Mail Order Companies Online

There are many companies that ship grass-fed meats and wild-raised fish to consumers nationwide.

For meat visit:

www.eatwild.com or www.uswellnessmeats.com

For poultry visit:

www.peacefulpastures.com or www.whiteegretfarm.com

For uncontaminated wild fish visit:

www.vitalchoice.com or www.ecofish.com

Other Resources

www.organicconsumers.org and www.factoryfarm.org

Meal Ideas

Good clean sources of protein are invaluable to the body. One cannot overcome illness nor achieve optimal health without using adequate amounts of good protein. The following ideas and recipes will help you incorporate different protein sources into your diet.

Breakfast:
- ✓ free-range eggs – poached, over easy, scrambled
- ✓ omelets with vegetables
- ✓ yogurt or kefir topped with fresh fruit, nuts, or seeds
- ✓ dinner leftovers
- ✓ whole grain toast with nut butter

Recipes:
- ✓ Egg Bake, page 156
- ✓ Egg Sandwich, page 156
- ✓ Yogurt-seed Surprise, page 158

Lunch:
- ✓ meat or fish topped salads
- ✓ cheese or egg topped salads
- ✓ chili or soups – grass-fed meat or vegetarian bean style
- ✓ turkey, beef, fish, or bean taco salad

✓ beans or quinoa added to salads or soups (quinoa is a grain source of protein)

Recipes:

✓ Chicken-Honey Mustard Salad, page 161

✓ Crazy Kim's Chicken Chili, page 165

✓ Crockpot Chili, page 167

✓ Turkey Taco Salad, page 172

Snacks:

✓ hummus and vegetables

✓ bean dips and spreads

✓ hard boiled eggs

Recipes:

✓ Deviled Eggs, page 155

✓ Hummus Dip, page 185

Dinner:

✓ free-range chicken dishes

✓ grass-fed meat dishes

✓ wild salmon or other wild-raised fish

✓ bean, rice, and vegetable dishes

Recipes:

- ✓ Creamy Chicken and Basil, page 166
- ✓ Juicy Hamburgers, page 168
- ✓ Pineapple Salsa Salmon, page 169
- ✓ Sloppy Lentils, page 170
- ✓ Super Sloppies (Sloppy Joe Style), page 171

5

Nuts and Seeds

Nuts and Seeds

Frequently Asked Questions

What are the nutritional benefits of nuts and seeds?

Nuts and seeds grow from plants and trees and are full of vitamins, minerals, antioxidants, phytochemicals, and phytosterols. Furthermore, nuts are a good source of healthy fats that help to build healthy immune and nervous systems. Although high in calories, the nutrients in nuts provide the body with a wonderful source of protein and a quick source of energy.

Nuts and seeds are some of the healthiest foods on the planet. For some of the many wholesome nutrients found in nuts, see Table 16.

Table 16: Healthy Nutrients in Nuts and Seeds

Almonds - more calcium than any other nut, copper, iron, potassium, phosphorus, riboflavin, vitamin E, zinc

Brazil Nuts – calcium, manganese, phosphorus, selenium, thiamin, zinc

Cashews – iron, magnesium, phosphorus, potassium, zinc

Hazelnuts – calcium, copper, iron, magnesium, phosphorus, potassium, manganese, thiamin

Pecans - monounsaturated oleic acid, calcium, iron, magnesium, phosphorus, potassium, selenium, zinc

Pumpkin Seeds - iron, phosphorus, potassium, riboflavin, thiamin

Cardiovascular disease is the number one killer for adults in the United States. Nuts have been shown in numerous studies to prevent heart disease.[1] [2] Also, hypertension has shown improvement with the use of nuts in the diet. Other illnesses which have been improved by consuming nuts are diabetes[3] and fatigue states.[4]

Due to the higher fat content of nuts, one criticism is that nuts may adversely affect cholesterol and lipid levels. However, nut consumption has been shown to lower elevated cholesterol levels and improve fatty acid profiles.[5] [6] Our experience is that nuts can be used to help improve the lipid profile in patients.

Are there any nuts or seeds to avoid?

Be wary of nuts with partially hydrogenated oils (e.g., soybean oil) which are an unnecessary source of harmful trans fat. Such nuts have no nutritional value. In addition, nuts that have been roasted are often topped with processed and refined salt, which can contain aluminum. You can roast nuts and seeds yourself and use natural Celtic Sea Salt. (For more information about unrefined salt, see Chapter 6, "Salt".)

Nuts also contain enzyme inhibitors and can be hard on the body to digest in raw form. We recommend preparing nuts by soaking overnight and roasting/dehydrating before eating (See Table 17). Soaking will decrease some of the enzyme inhibitors and also allow more of the nutrients of the nuts to become available to you.

Table 17: How to Dehydrate/Roast Nuts

1. Soak raw nuts overnight in large bowl with 2-3 teaspoons of Celtic Sea Salt and water. (Add more or less salt to taste.)

2. Strain.

3. Arrange nuts on cookie sheet and place in oven and cook at 150-175 degrees overnight or until dry. You can also use a dehydrator for drying.

Simple Diet Suggestions and Replacements

Nuts and seeds are best bought in their raw form (preferably organic) in packages, and not from bulk service bins where they may not be as fresh. Keep in mind that many of the prepackaged nut mixes can sometimes contain ingredients that are not as healthy. Be sure to look for and avoid products with added hydrogenated oils, additives, and excess salt.

Suggestion #1: Avoid commercially packaged nut mixes that have unnecessary salt, flavorings, and processed vegetable oils.

Replacement: Buy fresh, raw nuts, preferably in packages, and make up your own nut mixes.

Suggestion #2: Avoid roasted and salted nuts sold in packages at the grocery store.

Replacement: Buy raw nuts that you can soak in good quality sea salt and then dehydrate them yourself. (See Table 17, page 91)

Meal Ideas

Fresh nuts provide a wealth of nutrients for the body. Nuts can provide a source of quick energy before exercise. Furthermore, we suggest that nuts be added to the diet as a healthy snack alternative that both children and adults will learn to love. The following are some simple ideas for including nuts and seeds in the diet.

Breakfast:
- ✓ walnuts or pecans added to pancake or waffle mixes
- ✓ flax or sunflower seeds mixed in yogurt

Recipes:
- ✓ Yogurt-Seed Surprise, page 158

Lunch:
- ✓ nut butter sandwiches
- ✓ salad topped with almonds, cashews, or walnuts
- ✓ cashews, walnuts, or sesame seeds in vegetable dishes

Recipes:
- ✓ Almond Butter Sandwich, page 159
- ✓ Coconut Balsamic Salad, page 162

Snack:
- ✓ homemade nut mixes
- ✓ apples or pears topped with nut butter
- ✓ celery topped with nut butter

Recipes:

- ✓ Almighty Almonds Trail Mix, page 188
- ✓ Nuts for Chocolate Trail Mix, page 188
- ✓ Pecan Surprise Trail Mix, page 188

Dinner:

- ✓ nut crusted chicken dishes
- ✓ nuts added to your stir fry or curry dishes

Recipes:

- ✓ Vegetable Rice Stir Fry, page 173

Dessert:

- ✓ nut butter crusts
- ✓ nut toppings
- ✓ nut butter frosting

Recipes:

- ✓ Almond Butter-Coconut Crust, page 174
- ✓ Apple Bars, page 175
- ✓ Chocolate-Fudgy Frosting, page 178
- ✓ Cocoa-nut Milk Pudding Bars, page 179
- ✓ Nutty Fruit Cobbler, page 180

[1] Am. J. Clin. Nutr. 1999 Sep;70(3 Suppll):500-503
[2] Arch. Intern. Med. 2002. June 24;162(12):1382-7
[3] Int. J. Vitam. Nutr. Res. 2002 Oct;72(5):341
[4] Int. J. Obes. Relat. Metab. Disord. 2002. Aug;26(8):1129
[5] Am.F. Clin. Nutr. 2002 Nov;76(5):1000
[6] J.Nutr. 2001. Sep;131 (9):2275

6

Salt

Salt

Frequently Asked Questions

Do we need salt in our diet?

Yes, life itself is not possible without salt for humans, animals, and even plants. Throughout history, salt has been viewed as a valuable commodity. The Bible has several references to salt. Salt is commonly referred to as sodium chloride, the two main electrolytes found in all salt products. However, there is a vast difference in the quality of salt products. It is impossible to achieve your optimal health in a salt-deficient environment. In fact, a recent study found that higher salt intake was tied to longevity.[1]

What types of salt are available?

There are two salt products commonly available: unrefined natural salt that contains many valuable minerals, and refined table salt that is contaminated with aluminum and may exacerbate many chronic illnesses.

What is the most common salt sold in stores?

The most common salt found in grocery stores is table salt, which is refined white salt and is very fine. Table salt is 99.9% sodium chloride. It contains additives such as iodine, which was added to salt to prevent goiter. What is not as well known is that refined table salt also contains sugar (stabilizes iodine and used as an anti-caking agent) and aluminum. Refined table salt provides little nutritional value and should be avoided.

What is unrefined salt?

Unrefined salt is the only salt that retains its nutrient content. Unrefined salt, such as Celtic Sea Salt, preserves the vital balance of the ocean minerals. We have found Celtic Sea Salt a particularly useful form of salt. It contains over 80 minerals that the body needs to optimize its function, as shown below.

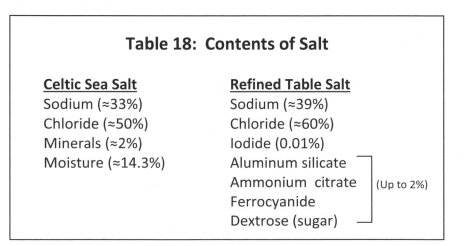

Table 18: Contents of Salt

Celtic Sea Salt
Sodium (≈33%)
Chloride (≈50%)
Minerals (≈2%)
Moisture (≈14.3%)

Refined Table Salt
Sodium (≈39%)
Chloride (≈60%)
Iodide (0.01%)
Aluminum silicate ⎤
Ammonium citrate ⎥ (Up to 2%)
Ferrocyanide ⎥
Dextrose (sugar) ⎦

How can you tell if salt is unrefined?

On the package it may say unrefined or unprocessed but, most importantly, unrefined salt often has a pink, grayish or a darker color to it and will also be moist. Refined salt, on the other hand, is usually white in color, as it has been bleached. We recommend that you use only unrefined salt in all of your recipes.

What are the benefits of unrefined salt?

The benefits of unrefined, natural salt are many. Table 19 lists some of these benefits. Refined salt (table salt) provides none of these benefits. If you have congestive heart failure or severe hypertension, your salt level may need to be monitored. We suggest you work with a holistic physician knowledgeable about natural products. For more information on the benefits of unrefined salt, we refer the reader to *Salt Your Way to Health, 2nd Edition* (Medical Alternatives Press: 1.888.647.5616).

Table: 19: Benefits of Unrefined Salt

- Alkalinizing agent (raises pH in the body)
- Balances blood sugar
- Helps relax the body for sleep
- Improves brain function
- Prevents muscle cramps
- Prevents varicose veins
- Prevents osteoporosis
- Regulates blood pressure (if adequately hydrated)
- Thins mucous

What are some sources of unrefined salt?

There are many sources of healthy, unrefined salt available for consumption. Table 20 lists just some of these sources.

Table 20: Sources of Unrefined Salt

- Bali Sea Salt
- Celtic Sea Salt from Brittany, France
- Eden Sea Salt, from France
- Halen Mon Pure Sea Salt, from Britain
- Hawaiian Red Alaea Salt
- Himalayan Crystal Salt
- Krystal Salt, from the Himalayas
- Redmond Real Salt, from Utah

Simple Diet Suggestions and Replacements

Salt is one of the most important nutrients for the body. Salt has been vilified by the media and many physicians for causing hypertension and other chronic health disorders. Those criticizing salt have no knowledge of the difference between unrefined and refined salt. It is important to include healthy unrefined salt in your diet and to avoid refined table salt.

Suggestion #1: Avoid commercially canned foods that often contain unnecessary and unnatural salt and flavorings.

Replacement: Buy fresh or frozen foods and season them yourself with unrefined salts such as those listed in Table 20, page 102.

Suggestion #2: Avoid common table salt in your home and at restaurants.

Replacement: Always have unrefined salt on hand at home for seasoning and cooking. Try carrying a small package of unrefined salt with you when going to a restaurant.

Meal Ideas

Refined salt should be avoided in the diet whenever possible and never intentionally added to foods. There are plenty of alternatives for seasoning and improving the taste of foods. Unrefined salt will bring out the natural flavors in your recipes.

Breakfast:
- ✓ pinch of unrefined salt in some water upon waking
- ✓ unrefined salt in the water for poaching eggs or on eggs
- ✓ unrefined salt in pancake, muffin, or other recipes

Lunch:
- ✓ unrefined salt on salads (keeps salads crisp)
- ✓ unrefined salt in soups and broths

Snacks:
- ✓ unrefined salt in dips and spreads
- ✓ pinch of unrefined salt in water to replenish after sports or working out (may help with cramps)
- ✓ unrefined salt on popcorn and other snacks

Recipes:
- ✓ Guacamole Dip, page 184
- ✓ Popcorn, page 189
- ✓ Zucchini Dip, page 187

Dinner:

- ✓ unrefined salt on meats for flavor or in marinades
- ✓ unrefined salt over vegetable dishes

Desserts:

- ✓ unrefined salt in cream when whipping it
- ✓ unrefined salt in egg whites for beating faster and higher

Recipes:

- ✓ Baked Custard, page 177

[1] Lancet. 3.14.1998;351:781-5

7

Making Children's Favorites Healthier

Making Children's Favorite Foods Healthier

Frequently Asked Questions

Why is it important to feed children healthy foods?

To allow your children the greatest opportunity for optimal health, it is important to supply them with the cleanest, highest quality foods. These foods will provide sources of vitamins, minerals, enzymes, amino acids, and other nutrients. A simple "balanced diet" is no longer sufficient due to the overabundance of highly refined and manufactured foods. Teach children the importance of good nutrition when they are young so they create healthy habits for the future. Emphasize the fact that processed foods, sugars, and soft drinks add zero nutrition to their diet, and that their use may even lead to health problems. Processed foods also make it less likely that they will eat the foods that contain essential nutrients they need for proper growth and development.

How can I feed my child healthier foods?

Replacing processed foods and implementing more whole foods can seem like a daunting task, especially in today's society. The processed food industries spend millions and sometimes billions of dollars on marketing highly processed, appealing junk foods in fun-looking packages to children. It is important, to make the time for, and put the energy into, meals and food preparation. Including children in food preparation often makes them more willing to sit down and eat those foods. (See Chapters 8 and 9 for shopping tips and Section IV for meal planning tips.) Although challenging at first, in order to eat good food, someone has to do some cooking (Remember, children love to be helpers!) Meals do not have to be gourmet, but a few extra minutes here and there can go a long way towards healthier meals. Children will learn good habits to carry into adulthood and even into their own family lives. The more you practice, the more efficient you will become. If your children are healthier, you may even save on doctors visits.

My child likes certain foods, can these be made healthier?

Yes, some of the "favorites" that children like (e.g., macaroni, chocolate cake, and grilled cheese, to name a few) will become healthier simply by making them at home with little or no processed food, and by using fresh ingredients that are safer for growing children's bodies as well as for your own. Most of the "favorites" in children's diets don't have to come from a can or a box, but can be made in your own kitchen.

Are there any healthy snacks I can feed my child?

Yes, there are many healthy choices for feeding your child at snack time. Look for fresh and unprocessed foods such as fruits and vegetables. Other ideas include fruit and cheese kabobs, carrots with ranch or hummus dip, apples or celery with nut butter or cream cheese, hard boiled eggs, yogurt, homemade muffins or cookies, trail mix, cheese and crackers, popcorn, and applesauce. For more kid-friendly recipes other than what is found in this book visit www.sherylshenefelt.com/shopwithsheryl. Items you want to avoid when purchasing snack foods include high fructose corn syrup, artificial colors and flavors, partially hydrogenated oils, trans fats, artificial sweeteners, and excessive sugar. Making snacks at home is the best way to ensure healthy ingredients and although they may take a bit more time, our children our worth it!

Simple Diet Suggestions and Replacements

Recipes are ideally made with the most natural ingredients possible, while being careful to avoid unnecessary flavorings, colorings, and preservatives. In addition, buy organics whenever possible to avoid pesticides that can be detrimental to a growing child's body. (For more on shopping, see Chapter 8, "Foods to Eat and Foods to Avoid" and for more on organics, see Section II, "Organic and Local Buying Tips".)

Suggestion #1: Avoid canned fruits and vegetables which have unnecessary sugars and salt.

Replacement: Fresh or frozen fruits and vegetables. Choose organic whenever possible to avoid unnecessary toxins.

Suggestion #2: Avoid white flour and white sugar breads, cookies, cakes, and other processed foods with little nutrient value.

Replacement: Look for whole grains and items without hydrogenated oils or high fructose corn syrup.

Suggestion #3: Avoid heating foods in the microwave since minerals, vitamins, and nutrients are reduced or altered (not to mention the other dangers that have been shown with microwaves).

Replacement: Use your stove top or regular cooking oven. A great investment is a toaster oven that can heat foods quickly and almost as easily as a microwave. Use broths to moisten foods and add flavor when reheating.

Suggestion #4: Avoid sugary sports drinks. Most sports drinks contain between 13 and 19 grams of sugar per 8 oz. serving. This is equivalent to approximately 3 to 5 packets of sugar!

Replacement: Drink good quality, filtered water regularly. A good rule of thumb is to take your body weight and divide it by two and that is how many ounces of water you should drink daily. For added electrolytes after a long workout try drinking coconut water. One cup-full of coconut water contains more electrolytes than most sports drinks and more potassium than a banana.

Meal Ideas

The following ideas include choosing more whole foods and possibly some extra preparation time. The more often vegetables can be hidden or added to a recipe unbeknownst to the child, the better! Some ideas are given in this section along with some recipes to give you a starting point that can be altered to fit your child's tastes or desires.

Breakfast:
- ✓ homemade muffins topped with butter
- ✓ homemade waffles with real maple syrup
- ✓ homemade French toast using free-range eggs

Recipes:
- ✓ Carrot Spice Muffins, page 152
- ✓ Cinnamon Waffles, page 153
- ✓ French Toast, page 157

Lunch:
- ✓ sandwiches with nut butters and berries or jam
- ✓ grilled cheese
- ✓ homemade macaroni and cheese
- ✓ homemade cheesy beef and macaroni

Recipes:

- ✓ Almond Butter Sandwich, page 159
- ✓ Cheese Quesadillas, page 159
- ✓ Cheesy Macaroni Dish, page 160
- ✓ Cheesy Beef and Macaroni, page 161

Snacks:

- ✓ homemade hummus with carrots or celery
- ✓ homemade popcorn topped with butter or coconut oil
- ✓ homemade salsa

Recipes:

- ✓ Hummus Dip, page 185
- ✓ Popcorn, page 189
- ✓ Simply Salsa, page 187

Dinner:

- ✓ homemade sloppy joe
- ✓ hamburgers and homemade fries
- ✓ homemade tacos
- ✓ homemade pizza (hide vegetables under the cheese!)

Recipes:

- ✓ Juicy Hamburgers, page 168
- ✓ Mini Muffin Pizzas, page 164
- ✓ Super Sloppies (Sloppy Joe Style), page 171

- ✓ Sweet Potato Fries, page 183
- ✓ Turkey Taco Salad (substitute taco shells), page 172

Desserts:
- ✓ homemade chocolate cake
- ✓ homemade chocolate pudding
- ✓ homemade cookies using natural sweeteners

Recipes:
- ✓ Chocolate Brownie Cake, page 178
- ✓ Cocoa-nut Milk Pudding, page 179

8

Foods to Eat and Foods to Avoid

Foods to Eat and Foods to Avoid

When grocery shopping, it is important to look at the ingredients on packages and food items before purchasing. Generally, if you cannot pronounce it, it probably isn't safe to eat. Many chemicals can be listed under a variety of names. If you have never heard of it, look it up or, better yet, avoid it altogether just to be safe!

FOODS TO EAT:

Buy whole, fresh foods only

Read labels carefully and look mostly for foods that contain only one or very few ingredients. Also, look for the word "whole" before the first ingredient on the label or ingredient list. Fresh food is more nutritious than frozen and frozen is better than canned. Always check for expiration dates on the label.

Produce

Buying fresh fruits and vegetables is a big part of having a healthy diet. Moreover, organic produce is much healthier and nutritious than non-organic produce. Ideally, all produce should be fresh, ripe, in season, and locally grown. Look for a local farmers' market or food co-op, or find the organic section at your grocery or health food store. Color counts — bring home an entire rainbow of colorful fruits and vegetables. (See "Organic and Local Buying Tips" in The Tips Section, page 199). A great video can be viewed online at www.storewars.org.

Poultry

Poultry should be organic (preferably free-range), antibiotic-free and hormone-free. Avoid meats from factory farms. More on factory farms can be found online at www.factoryfarm.org. Always look to support local farmers. Visit www.localharvest.org to find a farmer near you.

Seafood

Fish can be a great protein and is very rich in Omega-3 fatty acids, however, most fish is now contaminated with mercury, PCB's, and toxins, or unsustainably harvested. Buy mostly wild-caught fish or fish farmed in non-destructive and environmentally responsible ways. Fish should smell a bit like the sea, but fresh — it *should not* smell bad. Visit www.seafoodwatch.org for a more detailed guide to buying fish.

Meat

Buy only organic (preferably grass-fed), hormone-free, and antibiotic-free meats whenever possible. Many grocery stores carry grain-fed meats, which do not have the same wonderful benefits as grass-fed meats. See the benefits of grass-fed meat under resources at www.sherylshenefelt.com. Look for the specification that your meat is grass-fed or ask the butcher or farmer. Always look to support local farmers. Visit www.localharvest.org to find a farmer near you. A great video can be viewed online at www.meatrix.com.

Eggs

Ensure that you purchase eggs that are organic, antibiotic, and hormone-free. Preferably, you want to buy eggs from free-range hens so they have the proper ratios of Omega-3 and Omega-6 fatty acids. Eggs are the most complete protein and are a great source of long chain fats, EPA and DHA. We suggest you eat the whole egg to get the fat soluble vitamins and other nutrients which are found in the yolk of the egg.

FOODS TO AVOID:

Non-domestic produce

Fruits and vegetables raised in foreign countries are almost always sprayed with pesticides, preservatives, fecal fertilizers, or other harmful chemicals – like most non-organic foods from the U.S.

Most fish and seafood

Virtually all seafood, whether from fresh or salt water, is now contaminated with toxic metals and dangerous chemicals. Farm-raised seafood is the least healthy and often the most contaminated. In addition, many fish are non-sustainably harvested. Larger fish species are generally far more contaminated than smaller species. Warm water species are less safe than those from cold water. If you are pregnant, it is usually advisable to avoid seafood altogether. If you do eat fish, ensure the product is wild-caught or farmed from a source you trust.

Food with additives

Avoid purchasing foods with labels listing additives, colors, preservatives, emulsifiers, thickeners, anti-caking agents, bulking agents, flavorings, added seasonings or sauces, or chemical names you do not know or cannot pronounce.

Non-whole and processed foods

Avoid or limit products with more than one ingredient. These are NOT whole foods. Look for "100%", then carefully read what that 100% actually is. Breads and pasta are actually processed foods; whole, un-ground grains and sprouted grains are always healthier. If you must buy breads or pasta, look for the word "whole" or "sprouted" when the label describes the grains they came from. In general, avoid most packaged foods as these tend to have multiple unnecessary ingredients and additives.

Trans fats and hydrogenated fats

These particular fats are the "bad fats" that should be strictly avoided. Many items falsely imply they are trans fat-free yet still have hydrogenated oils in them. This is unfortunately because the government considers items to be trans fat-free if there is less than 0.5 grams of trans fat per serving.

MSG (monosodium glutamate)

MSG is a chemical used as a flavor enhancer in foods. It makes mediocre foods taste good. It may be disguised under names such as seasonings, spices, hydrolyzed proteins, soy protein isolate, or bouillon, just to name a few. This additive is extremely toxic to the nervous system and is known as a neurotoxin. More information can be found in the book *Excitotoxins: The Taste That Kills*, by Russell Blaylock.

Artificial sweeteners (e.g., aspartame, Splenda)

These are non-foods and they trick the body into thinking it is getting something sweet, which ultimately can create imbalance in the body. In addition, this type of sweetener has extremely toxic side effects. It is commonly found in fast foods, "fat-free" products, "sugar-free" products, diet soda, gums, ice creams, etc.

Genetically modified foods

Genetically modified (GM) foods may look and feel the same as conventional foods, but they are drastically (and possibly harmfully) different. Any item that is not organic may be genetically modified. Be aware of and avoid the most common GM foods, which include soy, corn, canola, and cotton. More information on GM foods can be found in the book *Seeds of Deception: Exposing Industry and Government Lies About the Safety of the Genetically Engineered Foods You're Eating*, by Jeffrey M. Smith.

Foods to Eat and Foods to Avoid List

Print this FREE online at www.sherylshenefelt.com/shopwithsheryl

	IDEAL	NEUTRAL	AVOID
M E A T	**Grass-fed, organic and antibiotic/hormone free** meat, like lamb, beef, wild game, goat, organ meat, and poultry.	Bacon, hot dogs, sausage, and lunch meats that are **free of nitrates, nitrites, hormones, antibiotics, and MSG.**	Commercial sausage and lunch meats, smoked meats, imitation or soy meats, and any meat from animals bred in confinement or that were exposed to antibiotics or hormones.
F I S H	**Fish that is fresh and caught wild from the ocean.** Fish that is not **over fished** or **destructively fished** and is **the least contaminated.** Best types include Arctic Char, wild Alaskan salmon, sardines, anchovies, Dungeness and stone crab, Pacific halibut, clams, mussels, oysters, herring, lobster (CA, FL), tuna, mussels, pink shrimp, and U.S. farmed: tilapia, rainbow trout, scallops (farmed).	Cod (Pacific), blue and U.S. king crab, Maine lobster, mahi-mahi, sablefish/black cod, sole (Pacific), northern shrimp, tilapia, tuna light and salmon canned in spring water, canned sardines, and whitefish acceptable in moderation, due to contamination from DDT, PCBs, and mercury.	Fish that is contaminated or overfished: cod (imported), grouper, orange roughy, sea bass, red snapper, swordfish, shark, tilefish, catfish, farmed salmon, fish that is canned in vegetable oils, fried fish, frozen fish sticks.

	IDEAL	NEUTRAL	AVOID
S T O C K S	Stocks from **grass-fed and/or organic** beef, chicken, turkey and fish.	**Organic** boxed or canned stocks.	Bouillon cubes.
E G G S	**Organic** eggs from **free-range** ducks or chickens, preferably from a local farmer. **Fertile** eggs have more nutrients.	**Organic, high omega-3** eggs from **free-range** or **cage-free** chickens.	Commercial eggs or **imitation** eggs (Egg Beaters).
N U T S & S E E D S	**Raw, organic nuts or seeds** and nut or seed products like almonds, walnuts, pistachios, pecans, cashews, nut butters **in their own oil** and soaked/dehydrated first is ideal. Sun butter, sunflower and pumpkin seeds, macadamia nuts, pine nuts, **coconut and coconut products** like milk or cream.	Nuts and seeds that are **not raw** or that are **dry-roasted**.	Nuts in **soy oil**, nut or seed butters that contain sugar or **hydrogenated oils**, and most **canned** nuts (including honey-roasted peanuts).

	IDEAL	NEUTRAL	AVOID
L E G U M E S	**Beans/Legumes** like lentils or beans (black, adzuki, kidney, garbanzo, pinto, and white). Preferably organic. **Fermented** soy like miso, tempeh, natto.	**Canned** beans/legumes and Valencia peanuts.	**Unfermented** soy, soy protein isolate, and hydrolyzed soy protein.
V E G E T A B L E S	**Non-starchy** vegetables like asparagus, kale, kohlrabi, Swiss chard, and cultured vegetables like sauerkraut. **Preferably organic, locally grown, in season.**	**Starchy** vegetables like carrots, potatoes, parsnips or corn, **frozen** vegetables, and canned tomatoes. **Preferably organic, locally grown, in season.**	**Canned** vegetables, **instant** mashed potatoes, and **pasteurized** veggies like pickles.
F R U I T S	Fruits that have a **low glycemic** index such as berries, apples, plums, oranges. **Preferably organic, locally grown, in season.**	**Higher glycemic** fruits, **frozen** fruits, **dried** fruits, or fruit leather. **Preferably organic, locally grown, in season.**	Fruits that contain **salt, additives, or preservatives**, fruit snacks, juice concentrate, and canned fruit.

	IDEAL	NEUTRAL	AVOID
F A T S A N D O I L S	Healthy fats and oils, which include **cold-pressed, extra virgin, and organic** items stored in a **dark container**. Organic butter (preferably grass-fed), ghee, extra virgin coconut oil, palm oil, extra virgin, cold pressed, olive oil, flax oil, high-vitamin butter oil (x-factor oil), and cod liver oil (from quality source).	**If in a dark container, cold-pressed, high oleic** safflower or sunflower oils, sesame or peanut oils in moderation. Also, grocery store butter, vegetable shortening made from palm, coconut or sesame oils, lard from **pastured, organic** pigs.	Oils exposed to **high heat, pressure, oxygen or light and/or containing chemicals**. Oils in clear bottles such as processed canola oil, commercial vegetable oils (soy, corn, cottonseed, safflower, sunflower), margarine, anything **partially hydrogenated**, shortening, and any spreads **containing vegetable oils or trans fats**.
B E V E R A G E S	**Filtered water**. **Raw** vegetable and fruit juices, coconut milk or water (kefired), herbal teas, and **naturally fermented** drinks like Kombucha.	**Bottled water, fresh-pressed** fruit juices, **organic** wine (sulfite-free), organic coffee and **un-pasteurized, microbrewed** beer.	Sodas, juice **concentrate**, Kool-Aid, **chlorinated or fluoridated** water, **diet** beverages, and hard alcohol.

	IDEAL	NEUTRAL	AVOID
G R A I N S	**Gluten-free** grains such as quinoa, millet, amaranth, buckwheat, brown rice, or **sprouted bread or sourdough** bread. wheat, spelt, kamut, oats, barley and rye may be tolerable if soaked and no gluten intolerance.	**Stone-ground, organic, 100% whole wheat** breads, hot breakfast cereals, pasta, crackers, spelt, wheat, kamut, oats, tortillas, and corn chips all that are **free of MSG, soy flour, corn syrup, or hydrogenated oils.**	**White flour products** including rice, breads, and pastas, cold breakfast cereals, granola, instant oatmeal, rice cakes, puffed grains, instant rice, or bread that **contains hydrogenated oils or soy flour.**
S W E E T E N E R S	**Nutrient rich, natural** sweeteners like raw honey, black strap molasses, maple syrup, and stevia. Also, sucanat, maple sugar, coconut palm sugar and date sugar.	**Minimally processed** sweeteners like beet sugar or sugar alcohols such as sorbitol and xylitol. Also, Lakanto and Lo Han alternate sweeteners.	**Highly processed, genetically modified** sweeteners that are lacking nutrients and can be toxic. These include corn syrup, white sugar, brown sugar and artificial sweeteners like aspartame (NutraSweet) and sucralose (Splenda). Agave nectar is also a highly processed sweetener.

	IDEAL	NEUTRAL	AVOID
D A I R Y	**Whole** milk and **raw or fresh** milk and cheese from **organic, grass-fed** cows or goats, organic plain yogurt, kefir and cream from whole milk.	**Low-heat pasteurized, non-homogenized** organic dairy from **grass-fed** cows or goats, plain yogurt or kefir, and rice, almond, or oat milks (preferably homemade).	**Processed or artificial** dairy products that have been **ultra-pasteurized or contain MSG (includes soy).** These include low fat and skim dairy, powdered milk, sweetened yogurts, NutraSweet yogurts, soy milk or cheese, ice cream, soy ice cream, imitation creamer, processed cheeses (including singles, sprays and spreads with additives), boxed milks, and canned whipped cream.
S P I C E S	**Unrefined** salt (e.g., Celtic sea salt) and **fresh herbs.**	**Dried** herbs, **un-iodized** sea salt	**Irradiated** spices, **iodized** salt, and **MSG** containing spices.

	IDEAL	NEUTRAL	AVOID
C O N D I M E N T S	**Raw or organic condiments** like ketchup **without corn syrup**, broths made from bones, **naturally fermented** soy sauce, apple cider vinegar, and sauerkraut free of vinegar.	Safflower oil mayonnaise and any sauces that **contain natural ingredients and have no MSG or corn syrup.** Low-heat processed whey protein from grass-fed cows	Mayonnaise containing **soy or canola oils,** any sauces containing **soy, MSG, or high-fructose corn syrup,** hydrolyzed proteins, and **denatured** whey protein.

9

What to Buy at the Grocery Store

Shopping Tips

When grocery shopping, it is important to look at the ingredients on packages and food items before purchasing. The following are some key questions to keep in mind. Remember, healthy food is not found in boxes, bags, cans, or packages, but is preferably obtained from your local farmer or farmers' markets, and is then prepared at home.

Can you pronounce it and do you know what it is?

Generally, if you cannot pronounce it, it probably isn't safe to eat. Many chemicals can be listed under a variety of names. If you have never heard of it, look it up. Make sure it is a food and something safe to ingest.

Can you make the item yourself?

Why not make the item yourself so you will know exactly what ingredients you are putting in. It will probably taste better anyway, and it will allow you to use better quality ingredients, including organic ingredients. For example, hydrogenated oils could be replaced with butter or coconut oil, and corn syrup could be replaced with natural sweeteners.

Is there a brand with fewer additives that could be substituted?

Check around and see if one of the other brands has fewer additives, or go to a health food store and see if there is a replacement. Avoid purchasing foods with labels listing additives, colors, preservatives, emulsifiers, thickeners, anti-caking agents, bulking agents, flavorings, added seasonings or sauces, or chemical names you don't know or can't pronounce. Most of the time, the product will taste better without the foreign ingredients. You may have to do some taste testing to find the brand you like best.

Can you buy it fresh (second best is frozen), rather than canned?

It is always a good idea to get foods in the freshest form possible. Raw fruits and vegetables would be the first choice, followed by frozen which contains more nutrient value than canned and definitely less additives. Ideally, all produce should be fresh, ripe, in season, and locally grown. Shopping at farmers' markets is always a good idea. Be sure to look for organic options which are a healthier and more nutritious choice. (For more on buying organic and local food, see Tips Section II)

Do you know the source or could you find a higher nutrient quality source?

Ask questions when grocery shopping, especially with prepared items or delicatessen items. Find out what ingredients were added, how long ago it was made, and even where the ingredients came from so you can determine the nutritional quality. Avoid items with multiple ingredients listed and choose those with just the one or two necessary items for that food.

Is the item coming from a foreign country?

Avoid foods grown outside of the United States (even frozen foods), because places such as Mexico, Central America, and South America may not have the same high standards as we do in the United States. Furthermore, even though certain toxic pesticides may be banned in the United States, we export them to other countries, and then get them shipped right back to us on the fruits and vegetables we import!

Do you know how the meat or fish was raised or the living conditions of the animals?

Buy only organic or free-range, hormone- and antibiotic-free meats whenever possible. Grass-fed beef is the best choice-- always try to support local farmers. When buying fish, avoid farm-raised fish and be sure the fish is fresh (wild fish is optimal). Some examples of questions to ask include: Is the fish farm-raised or wild? Are the eggs from free-range chickens? Are the cows grass-fed or grain-fed? Free-range and grass-fed are better choices since the food from a grass-fed animal will contain more vitamins and minerals and a healthier assortment of essential fatty acids as compared to grain-fed animals.

Does the product contain harmful hydrogenated oils, artificial sweeteners, or high fructose corn syrup?

Look for products that are free of hydrogenated oils, which often contain harmful trans fats. Safer choices would be items made with butter, coconut oil, and palm oil because those types of fats can withstand higher heats often used in processing. Also, avoid products with artificial sweeteners which are toxic to the body as well as high fructose corn syrup that, along with the excess sugar content, are often laden with other chemicals and additives. Choose foods made with natural sweeteners or buy the ingredients to make your own foods so you know what is in them.

Does the product contain genetically modified ingredients?

Genetically modified (GM) foods may look and feel the same as conventional foods, but they are drastically (and possibly harmfully) different. These types of foods have been altered by taking the genetic material (DNA) from one species and transferring it into another in order to obtain a desired trait. The

FDA does not require any safety testing or any labeling of GM foods, and introducing new genes into a fruit or vegetable may very well be creating unknown results such as new toxins, new bacteria, new allergens, and new diseases. Be aware of the most common GM foods, which include soy, corn, canola, and cotton. The only way to completely avoid genetically modified foods is to buy organic foods. More on genetic engineering can be found at www.seedsofdeception.com.

Suggested Brands

The following list includes grocery store items that the authors like (strictly opinions), although we want to make note that of course it is preferable to buy things from farms and not in boxes, bags, cans, or packages. To find local farmers visit www.localharvest.org. For more product suggestions and resources visit www.sherylshenefelt.com.

For those people just getting started toward making healthier choices, and even for those who have been on this path for some time now, we have compiled a list of items that we find to be good choices and without key harmful ingredients such as hydrogenated oils, high fructose corn syrup, soy, MSG, etc. We have also included a handy shopping check-list for you to take to the store with you. For those of you interested in raw milk and raw milk products, we refer you to www.realmilk.com to find a local farmer or you can purchase from www.organicpastures.com.

PRODUCE SECTION

In this area, it is important to look at the signs as well as the labels on the fruit. Sometimes you think you are buying organic and it turns out you grabbed the conventional ones that are right next to the organic section. The numbers on the labels actually stand for something and can be important as you select your food. Items containing 4-digits beginning with a 3 or a 4 are conventional. Items with 5-digits beginning with a 9 are organic. There are some common fruits and vegetables that are best bought organic due to the numerous toxic pesticides and herbicides used to grow them: apples, cherries, celery, grapes (imported), lettuce, nectarines, peaches, pears, potatoes, spinach, sweet bell peppers, and strawberries. On the other hand, there are also some fruits and vegetables that, if necessary, would be the safest to buy conventional: avocado, asparagus, banana, broccoli, cabbage, eggplant, kiwi, mango, onion, and pineapple.

Gluten-Free Note: The list below contains many items that are marked with a * if that brand offers gluten-free options. It is always a good idea to double check the labels because manufacturers change their ingredients sometimes several times throughout the year. Also, if you are strictly gluten-free, double-check to be sure that the item you are buying is not made in the same facility or on the same equipment as wheat or gluten products where cross-contamination can occur. For more on gluten-free eating, please refer to the authors' *The Guide to a Gluten-Free Diet*. In addition, if you are on a dairy-free diet, please refer to the authors' book *The Guide to a Dairy-Free Diet*.

FATS/OILS

- ✓ Butter - Kalona, Kerrygold*, Organic Valley Pastured*, Trader Joe's Sweet Cream*
- ✓ Coconut oil - Garden of Life or online: Omega Nutrition*, Tropical Traditions*, Wilderness Family Naturals*
- ✓ Coconut milk (organic, whole) – Native Forest, Thai Kitchen
- ✓ Flax oil - Barleans*
- ✓ Ghee – Purity Farms*
- ✓ Mayonnaise – Hain Safflower Oil
- ✓ Olive oil – Bionaturae*, Colavita*,
- ✓ Palm Oil – Jungle*

NUT BUTTERS

- ✓ Almond Butter - Maranatha Raw Products*
- ✓ Tahini – Maranatha Raw Products*
- ✓ Peanut Butter – Arrowhead Mills (Valencia peanuts)*

CANNED GOODS

- ✓ Beans – Eden*, Westbrae*
- ✓ Broth – Health Valley Organic Free Range Chicken Broth*, Shelton's
- ✓ Pizza Sauce – Eden*, Muir Glen*
- ✓ Spaghetti Sauce – Walnut Acres, Low Sodium*
- ✓ Sockeye Salmon – Bumble Bee*, Natural Sea*
- ✓ Soups – Amy's
- ✓ Tomatoes - Eden Organic*, Muir Glen*
- ✓ Tuna Fish –Crown Prince*, Natural Sea*, Trader Joe's Tongul tuna in water*

BAKING

- ✓ Baking Powder and Baking Soda– Bob's Red Mill (aluminum-free)*
- ✓ Chocolate Chips - Enjoy Life*, Sunspire
- ✓ Flours – Bob's Red Mill Stone Ground Flours (various types, some gluten-free)*, online www.organicsproutedflour.net

- ✓ Spices – Frontier or organic spices
- ✓ Sweeteners – Coconut palm sugar, Rapadura*, Really Raw Honey*, Shady Maple Farms Maple Syrup*, Sucanat*
- ✓ Vanilla – Frontier*

PASTA AND RICE

- ✓ Pasta – Eden Soba and Pasta, Tinkyada Organic Brown Rice Pastas*, Ezekiel Sprouted Spaghetti
- ✓ Rice – Lundberg Farms*

BREAD

- ✓ Bread, bagels, buns, English muffins – Alvarado Street Bakery Sprouted, Cybros Sprouted, Food for Life Sprouted
- ✓ Bread – Berlin Natural Bakery sourdough spelt, French Meadow Bakery European sourdough rye
- ✓ Gluten-Free Bread - Food for Life Millet* or Rice* or homemade versions
- ✓ Tortillas - Alvarado Street Bakery, Food for Life
- ✓ Gluten-Free Tortillas - Food for Life*

CEREAL

- ✓ Buckwheat – Bob's Red Mill Creamy Buckwheat Hot Cereal*
- ✓ Oats – Bob's Red Mill or Bob's Red Mill Gluten-Free *
- ✓ Dry cereal - Ezekiel

SNACKS

- ✓ Applesauce – Eden*, Woodstock Farms*
- ✓ Crackers - Ak-mak, Wasa
- ✓ Dried fruit – Newman's Own organic*
- ✓ Chips - Kettle Organic Chips, Lundberg Farms Organic Sea Salt Rice Chips*
- ✓ Rice crackers - Edward and Sons rice crackers*, San J *
- ✓ Popcorn – Eden organic*
- ✓ Various Snacks (recommended for occasional use only) – Annie's, Back to Nature, Late July

MEATS

- ✓ Bacon or turkey bacon without nitrites/nitrates - Applegate Farms*, Wellshire Farms*
- ✓ Sliced meat without nitrites/nitrates - Applegate Farms*
- ✓ Sausages and hot dogs without nitrites/nitrates - Applegate Farms*, Organic Prairie*, Shelton's*

DAIRY AND EGGS

- ✓ Cream –Organic Valley*, Trader Joe's*
- ✓ Cheese (Cow) – Organic Valley "Raw" Cheeses* or raw from cheese counters
- ✓ Cheese (Goat) – Mt. Sterling "Raw" Cheeses* or raw from cheese counters
- ✓ Dairy products (cottage cheese, sour cream, etc.) - Kalona*, Organic Valley Products*
- ✓ Milk (Low-Heat Pasteurized) – Kalona*
- ✓ Eggs – Farmer's Hen House*, Gold Circle Farms*, Organic Valley*, Trader Joe's Fertile*
- ✓ Yogurt (Buffalo) – Woodstock Water*
- ✓ Yogurt (Cow) - Brown Cow*, FAGE Total Classic Greek Yogurt*, Seven Stars Organic*, Stoneyfield*, Traders Point Creamery*, Trader Joe's Greek Style plain yogurt*, Thomas Creamery
- ✓ Yogurt and Kefir(Goat) - Redwood Hill*

DESSERTS

- ✓ Bars - Govinda's Bliss Bars*, Lara Bars*
- ✓ Chocolate – Dagoba*, Green and Black's*
- ✓ Cocoa - Dagoba*, Green and Black's*
- ✓ Vanilla Ice Cream (Cow) – Julie's*, Sibby's*, Stoneyfield*

- ✓ Vanilla Ice Cream (Goat) – LaLoo's*
- ✓ Coconut Milk Ice Cream – Coconut Bliss*, Purely Decadent*

CONDIMENTS

- ✓ Apple Cider Vinegar – Bragg's (Raw) *, Eden*
- ✓ Balsamic Vinegar - Bionaturae
- ✓ Ketchup – Annie's*, Muir Glen
- ✓ Mayonnaise – Hain Safflower Oil
- ✓ Mustard – Annie's*, Hain, Westbrae
- ✓ Rice Vinegar - Eden*
- ✓ Soy Sauce (Naturally Fermented)– Eden, San-J

FREEZER

- ✓ Frozen Fruit and Vegetables - Cascadian Farms*, Tree of Life*, Woodstock Farms*

BEVERAGES

- ✓ Kombucha – Synergy*, Buchi
- ✓ Rice Smoothie - Amazake*
- ✓ Sparkling Water – Gerolsteiner, San Pellegrino*, Perrier*
- ✓ Tea –Celestial Seasonings Organic, Yogi Organic

10

Recipes

Recipes

Breakfast Recipes (pages 152-158)

- ❖ Carrot Spice Muffins
- ❖ Cinnamon Waffles
- ❖ Date-Oat Bars
- ❖ Deviled Eggs
- ❖ Egg Bake
- ❖ Egg Sandwich
- ❖ French Toast
- ❖ Healthy Smoothie
- ❖ Yogurt-Seed Surprise

Lunch Recipes (pages 159-164)

- ❖ Almond Butter Sandwich
- ❖ Cheese Quesadillas
- ❖ Cheesy Macaroni Dish
- ❖ Cheesy Beef and Macaroni
- ❖ Chicken-Honey Mustard Salad
- ❖ Coconut Balsamic Salad
- ❖ Creamy Vegetable Bean Soup
- ❖ Lentil Sweet Potato Soup
- ❖ Mini Muffin Pizzas

Dinner Recipes (pages 165-173)

- ❖ Crazy Kim's Chicken Chili
- ❖ Creamy Chicken and Basil
- ❖ Crockpot Chili
- ❖ Juicy Hamburgers
- ❖ Pineapple Salsa Salmon
- ❖ Sloppy Lentils
- ❖ Super Sloppies (Sloppy Joe Style)
- ❖ Turkey Taco Salad
- ❖ Vegetable Rice Stir Fry

Dessert Recipes (pages 174-180)

- ❖ Almond Butter-Coconut Crust
- ❖ Apple Bars
- ❖ Applesauce Cake
- ❖ Baked Custard
- ❖ Chocolate Brownie Cake
- ❖ Chocolate-Fudgy Frosting
- ❖ Cocoa-nut Milk Pudding
- ❖ Cocoa-nut Milk Pudding Bars
- ❖ Nutty Fruit Cobbler

Vegetable Side Recipes (pages 181-183)

- ❖ Coconut Green Beans
- ❖ Ginger Quinoa Squash
- ❖ Lemon Tahini Kale
- ❖ Sweet Potato Fries

Dip and Salsa Recipes (pages 184-187)

- ❖ Guacamole Dip
- ❖ Hummus Dip
- ❖ Pineapple Chipotle Salsa
- ❖ Simply Salsa
- ❖ Zucchini Dip

Snack Recipes (pages 188-189)

- ❖ Almighty Almonds Trail Mix
- ❖ Nuts for Chocolate Trail Mix
- ❖ Pecan Surprise Trail Mix
- ❖ Popcorn

Spread Recipes (Page 190)

- ❖ Honey Coconut Butter Spread
- ❖ Strawberry Coconut Butter Spread
- ❖ Cinnamon Coconut Oil Spread

Note: Recipe ingredients with * are found at health food stores, but may be substituted with similar item. We suggest choosing organic for all ingredients in recipes if your budget allows.

Carrot Spice Muffins

2	cups brown rice flour* or spelt flour*
1½	cups whole, plain yogurt
2	teaspoons baking soda
1	teaspoon cinnamon
½	teaspoon sea salt
¼	teaspoon ground ginger
¼	teaspoon ground cloves
⅔	cup coconut oil, melted
⅔	cup Sucanat or coconut palm sugar*
2	free-range, organic eggs
1	teaspoon vanilla
1	cup carrots, grated
½	cup raisins or zante currants* (optional)

Servings: 22-24   Prep: 10 minutes   Cook: 18 minutes

Combine flour and yogurt in a large bowl and let soak overnight. Add baking soda and all spices to yogurt mixture and set aside. In a separate bowl, blend oil with Sucanat or coconut palm sugar. Add eggs, vanilla, and carrots and mix. Slowly add yogurt mixture to carrot mixture and stir until moistened. Add raisins or currants, if using. Fill well greased muffin pan (try using coconut oil) and bake at 300˚F for about 18 minutes. Delicious topped with butter for breakfast or anytime!

Serving Suggestions: *Top with Honey Coconut Butter, page 190, Cinnamon Coconut Oil Spread, page 190, or butter.*

Cinnamon Waffles

2   cups whole grain spelt or oat flour*
1⅔ cups whole, plain yogurt or kefir
3   free-range, organic eggs
1   tablespoon coconut oil, melted
1   tablespoon raw honey*
1   teaspoon baking soda
1   teaspoon sea salt
1   teaspoon cinnamon
¼   teaspoon nutmeg
1-2 tablespoons filtered water

Servings: 6-8   Prep: 10 minutes   Cook: 15 minutes

Combine spelt flour with yogurt or kefir and let soak overnight. Blend in remaining ingredients using a hand mixer, adding water to thin if necessary. Pour by spoonfuls onto waffle maker and heat through.

Serving Suggestions: *Top with Honey Coconut Butter, page 190, butter, maple syrup, fruit, or preserves.*

Date-Oat Bars

2½   cups rolled oats
1¾   cups whole, plain yogurt
1   pound pitted dates, chopped
½   cup organic butter
¼   cup raw honey*
⅔   cup pecans, chopped
1½   teaspoons vanilla
½   teaspoon cinnamon

Servings: 8-10   Prep: 20 minutes   Cook: 5 minutes

Combine oats and yogurt in small bowl, cover and let soak overnight. In small saucepan over medium heat, cook dates, butter, and honey for 4 to 5 minutes or until thickened, stirring constantly. Mix in soaked oat mixture, pecans, vanilla, and cinnamon.   Spread in buttered 9 X 13 inch Pyrex dish and chill for a couple hours before serving. Date-Oat Bars are meant to have a wet consistency to them.

Serving Suggestions: *Serve topped with fresh cream and/or chopped berries.*

Deviled Eggs

4   free-range, organic eggs
¼   teaspoon sea salt
2   tablespoons whole, plain yogurt or mayonnaise
2   teaspoons Dijon mustard
¼   teaspoon cayenne pepper (or to taste)

Servings: 4   Prep: 10 minutes   Cook: 15 minutes

Hard boil eggs by placing in cold water with ¼ teaspoon sea salt and bringing water to boil. Boil 10 minutes and let sit 2 minutes. Cover with cool water and let sit another 2 minutes. Peel eggs and cut in half. Remove yolks, place in bowl, and mash. Mix in other ingredients and then put a little of mixture into each egg white half.

Serving Suggestions: *To spice it up, add horseradish (especially with yogurt version). For decoration, sprinkle the eggs with paprika or parsley.*

Egg Bake

½   cup spinach, chopped
½   cup red pepper, chopped
¼   cup onion, chopped
6   free-range, organic eggs (lightly beaten)
1   cup feta cheese, crumbled
⅓   cup organic, heavy cream
½   teaspoon basil
¼   teaspoon oregano
½   teaspoon sea salt

Servings: 4-6   Prep: 15 minutes   Cook: 40 minutes

Chop all vegetables and set aside. In large bowl, beat eggs and combine with the cheese, cream, and spices. Mix in vegetables and then pour into a buttered 8 X 8 inch Pyrex dish. Bake at 300°F for 40 minutes or until firm and browned on top.

Serving Suggestions: *Serve with sour cream or Salsa, page 187.*

Egg Sandwich

2   teaspoons coconut oil
1   free-range, organic egg
1   piece sprouted, whole grain bread*
1   tablespoon organic butter
1   tablespoon cream cheese (optional)
1   pinch sea salt

Servings: 1   Prep: 5 minutes   Cook: 8 minutes

Heat pan over medium heat. Melt coconut oil and crack egg into pan. Cook egg 2-3 minutes until top of white has just begun to set. Flip and cook 1-2 more minutes ("over easy" style egg). While egg is cooking, toast the bread. Spread toasted bread with butter and cream cheese and place cooked egg on top. Sprinkle with sea salt and serve.

Serving Suggestions: *Serve with thinly sliced tomato.*

French Toast

1	tablespoon coconut oil
4	free-range, organic eggs (lightly beaten)
¼	cup organic heavy cream
1	teaspoon vanilla
¼	teaspoon nutmeg
6	slices sprouted, whole grain bread*

Servings: 3-4   Prep: 10 minutes   Cook: 10 minutes

Heat coconut oil in skillet over medium heat. Combine eggs, cream, vanilla, and nutmeg in square dish. Dip bread into egg mixture to cover both sides. Cook in skillet until lightly browned on both sides.

Serving Suggestions: *Top with Honey Coconut Butter, page 190, Cinnamon Coconut Oil Spread, page 190, butter, or maple syrup.*

Storage Suggestion: *Make in large batches and separate with waxed paper before storing. Store them in the freezer for quick reheating in the toaster.*

Healthy Smoothie

½   cup yogurt, kefir, or coconut milk*
½   cup filtered water
1   cup frozen fruit – mango, strawberries, etc
1   teaspoon kelp powder* (optional)
1   teaspoon cod liver oil* (optional)
1   raw free-range, organic egg yolk (optional)

Servings: 1-2   Prep: 10 minutes

Mix together in a blender until smooth and creamy.

Serving Suggestions: *Add raw honey to taste and serve chilled.*

Yogurt-Seed Surprise

1   cup whole, plain yogurt
¼   cup blueberries
2   tablespoons sunflower seeds
1   tablespoon organic maple syrup (to taste)

Mix all ingredients together and serve.

Servings: 1   Prep: 5 minutes

Serving Suggestions: *Serve with various fresh berries such as raspberries or strawberries instead of (or in addition to) blueberries.*

Lunch Recipes

Almond Butter Sandwich

2   pieces sprouted, whole grain bread*
1   tablespoon raw almond butter in its natural oil
½   cup chopped berries (or 1 tablespoon low-sugar jam)

Servings: 1   Prep: 5 minutes   Cook: 2 minutes

Spread bread with almond (or peanut) butter and add chopped berries (or low-sugar jam) and serve.

Serving Suggestions: *Toast the bread before making sandwich.*

Cheese Quesadillas

4   sprouted wheat tortillas*
2   tablespoons organic butter
2½ cups shredded raw cheese*
1   tablespoon coconut oil

Servings: 2   Prep: 10 minutes   Cook: 5 minutes

Butter the outsides of the tortillas. Place cheese on non-buttered side of tortilla and make a sandwich with two tortillas keeping butter sides facing out. Cook in coconut oil at medium-high heat, flipping once, until both sides are lightly browned and cheese is melted in the middle.

Serving Suggestions: *Add vegetables or meat to quesadilla. Great served with homemade Salsa, page 187.*

Cheesy Macaroni Dish

2   cups brown rice elbow pasta*
6   tablespoons of organic butter
1   cup whole, plain organic yogurt
½   teaspoon onion flakes
¼   teaspoon nutmeg
¼   teaspoon white pepper
¼   teaspoon black pepper
⅛   teaspoon sea salt
2   pinches dried mustard
1   cup organic chicken broth
¼   cup arrowroot powder
2   free-range, organic eggs (lightly beaten)
2   cups shredded raw sharp cheddar cheese*
⅓   cup Romano cheese, grated

Servings: 8   Prep: 25 minutes   Cook: 30 minutes

Preheat oven to 350°F. Cook pasta al dente style or 2 minutes less than time on package, drain and set aside. While pasta is cooking melt butter in a medium size pan. Add yogurt and spices and bring to slow boil. In small container, combine chicken broth with arrowroot powder and shake. Slowly pour broth mixture into pan with yogurt and continue stirring until it begins to thicken. Lightly beat eggs and add to mixture along with both of the cheeses and stir until melted. Add al dente pasta to cheese mixture until coated. Transfer to a greased 9 X 13 dish and spread evenly. Bake covered at 350°F for 15 minutes, remove cover and bake another 10 minutes or until bubbly all over. Broil 2-3 minutes until the top is lightly browned before serving.

Serving Suggestions: *Add dried bread crumb pieces, extra Romano cheese or sprinkle paprika and parsley on top before baking.*

Cheesy Beef and Macaroni

½   recipe Cheesy Macaroni Dish (see page 160, use leftovers!)
1   pound ground beef, browned
⅔   cup organic ketchup

Add ground beef and ketchup to ½ a recipe of Cheesy Macaroni and you have dinner for one more night!

Chicken-Honey Mustard Salad

¼   cup lemon juice
2   tablespoons Dijon mustard
2   tablespoons raw honey
1   clove garlic, minced
1   dash cayenne pepper (optional)
½   cup extra virgin olive oil
1   tablespoon cold-pressed flax oil
2   free-range, organic chicken breasts
2   tablespoons coconut oil
1   head green or red leaf lettuce
1   cucumber, chopped
1-2 hard boiled, organic eggs (chopped)

Servings: 3-4   Prep: 15 minutes   Cook: 15 minutes

To make dressing, combine lemon, mustard, honey, and garlic (and cayenne pepper, if using) in food processor. While processing, add olive oil in slow stream and then flax oil. Sauté chicken breasts in coconut oil over medium-high heat, cool and cut into cubes. Combine lettuce, cucumber, hard boiled eggs, and chicken, and serve with dressing.

Serving Suggestions: *Refrigerate dressing about 15 minutes before serving.*

Coconut Balsamic Salad

⅛   cup coconut milk
1½ tablespoons Balsamic vinegar
1   teaspoon Dijon mustard
½   teaspoon dried basil
¼   teaspoon sea salt
¼   cup extra virgin olive oil
½   tablespoon cold-pressed flax oil
1   head of romaine lettuce, washed and chopped
1   cup raw walnuts, chopped
½   cup feta cheese, crumbled
½   cup dried cranberries

Servings: 3-4   Prep: 15 minutes

To make salad dressing, combine coconut milk, vinegar, mustard, basil, and sea salt in food processor. While processing, add olive oil in slow stream and then flax oil. Combine lettuce, walnuts, feta, and cranberries, and serve with dressing.

Serving Suggestions: *Refrigerate dressing about 15 minutes before serving.*

Creamy Vegetable Bean Soup

3	cups red kidney beans (canned or cooked)
3	cups garbanzo beans (canned or cooked)
4	cups vegetable or chicken broth
3½	cups chopped or frozen vegetables (broccoli, zucchini, carrots)
1	cup tomato, diced
1	cup spinach, chopped
¾	cup onion, chopped
1	tablespoon tomato paste
4-5	cloves garlic, minced
1	teaspoon parsley
½	teaspoon sea salt
½	teaspoon pepper
¼	teaspoon basil
1	pint organic heavy cream

Servings: 6-8   Prep: 25 minutes   Cook: 3-4 hours

Drain and rinse beans before placing them into a crock pot. Add broth and the rest of the ingredients to the crock pot, except cream. Cover and cook on high-heat setting for 3-4 hours (or on low-heat setting for 6-8 hours). When the soup is finished, put half of the soup in a blender and puree it. Return to crock pot and add the cream. Cover and cook ½ hour more and serve.

Serving Suggestions: *Serve with cream on the side.*

Lentil Sweet Potato Soup

1   onion, chopped
2   tablespoons coconut oil
5   cups organic chicken broth (or water)
⅛   teaspoon cumin
⅛   teaspoon coriander
½   teaspoon turmeric
2   bay leaves
2   teaspoons sea salt (not as much if using broth)
1   cup red lentils (uncooked)
1   large sweet potato, chopped
4-5 carrots, chopped

Servings: 4   Prep: 20 minutes   Cook: 55 minutes

In a large pot, sauté onion in coconut oil until tender. Stir in broth and spices. Add lentils, sweet potato, and carrots and bring to boil. Skim froth at top, reduce heat, and simmer covered for about 50 minutes.

Serving Suggestions: *Serve with Carrot Spice muffins, page 152.*

Mini Muffin Pizzas

1   cup organic tomato sauce
¼   teaspoon each basil and oregano
3   sprouted, whole grain English muffins*
2½ cups raw cheddar cheese, shredded

Servings: 3   Prep: 15 minutes   Cook: 3-4 minutes

Heat the tomato sauce, basil, and oregano over medium-low heat. Cut muffins into halves and toast them. Spread muffins with tomato sauce mixture and sprinkle cheese on top. Put under broiler for 3-4 minutes, or until cheese is melted, and serve.

Serving Suggestions: *Sauté spinach or other vegetables and mix into tomato sauce. Vegetables can be hidden under the cheese!*

Crazy Kim's Chicken Chili

3	cups great northern white beans (canned or cooked)
4	free-range chicken breasts, chopped
½	cup onion, chopped
2	tablespoons coconut oil
4	cups organic chicken broth
1	teaspoon cumin
1	teaspoon chili powder
¼	cup green chilies, chopped

Servings: 4   Prep: 15 minutes   Cook: 40 minutes

Sauté chicken and onions in coconut oil until tender and chicken is cooked through. Drain and rinse beans and place half of them into the pot, mash, and then add remaining ingredients. Simmer 30 minutes and serve.

Serving Suggestions: *Serve with garnishes of sour cream, raw cheese, chopped onion.*

Creamy Chicken and Basil

4	free-range, organic chicken breasts
2	tablespoons coconut oil
1	cup organic heavy cream (or yogurt)
1	pinch sea salt
4	tablespoons organic butter
2	tablespoons fresh basil, chopped finely
1	tablespoon sea salt
1	teaspoon black pepper
1	cup organic chicken broth
2	tablespoons arrowroot*
1	cup spinach, chopped

Servings: 4   Prep: 15 minutes   Cook: 20 minutes

Sauté chicken in coconut oil about 4 minutes per side until almost fully cooked. Meanwhile, whip heavy cream and a pinch of sea salt with hand mixer until it begins to thicken. Pour whipped cream mixture along with butter, basil, salt, and pepper into pan and bring to just under a boil. Combine broth with arrowroot and mix to dissolve. Pour slowly into cream mixture and stir slowly until thickened. Add chicken and spinach to pan and heat until spinach softens and chicken is cooked through.

Serving Suggestions: *Serve over rice or quinoa.*

Crockpot Chili

3   cups kidney beans (canned or cooked)
1   pound grass-fed, organic, ground beef
3   cups diced tomatoes
⅓   cup tomato paste
½   cup organic beef broth
½   onion, diced
½   green or red pepper, diced (optional)
2   teaspoons chili powder
3   teaspoons cumin
Sea salt, pepper, cayenne to taste

Servings: 4   Prep: 15 minutes   Cook: 5-6 hours

Drain and rinse beans before placing them into a crock pot. Brown beef, drain, and add to crock pot. Add the rest of the ingredients and stir. Cover and cook in crock pot for 5-6 hours.

Serving Suggestions: *Serve with garnishes of sour cream, raw cheese, chopped onion, and/or jalapeno peppers.*

Juicy Hamburgers

1   pound grass-fed, organic ground beef
1   free-range, organic egg
2   dashes Worcestershire sauce
1   teaspoon each of sea salt and pepper
1   cup raw cheese*, thinly sliced
4   sprouted, whole grain hamburger buns

Servings: 4   Prep: 15 minutes   Cook: 15 minutes

Combine beef, egg, Worcestershire, salt and pepper in bowl and mash together until blended. Form into 4 hamburgers and grill to desired temperature. Top with raw cheese and let melt while still over heat.

Serving Suggestions*: Toast or grill sprouted, whole grain hamburger buns with butter and garlic on them. Serve with ketchup, mustard, lettuce, tomato, onion.*

Storage Suggestion:* Make in large batches and freeze in preformed patties separated by waxed paper. For a quick meal just remove from freezer and put on the grill!*

Pineapple Salsa Salmon

1   pound wild salmon
2   teaspoons coconut oil
2   wedges of lemon
2   cloves garlic, crushed
1   recipe Pineapple Chipotle Salsa (see page 186)

Servings: 4   Prep: 10 minutes   Cook: 20 minutes

Preheat oven to 350°F. Combine coconut oil, lemon, and garlic in small bowl.   Spread mixture over salmon and then bake at 350°F for 20 minutes, or to desired appearance. Top salmon with Pineapple Chipotle Salsa, page 186.

Serving Suggestions: *Serve with a side of cream or sour cream.*

Sloppy Lentils

1½ cups lentils (uncooked)
3   cups filtered water
1   tablespoon lemon juice
½   cup green pepper, chopped
½   cup onion, chopped
3   cups tomatoes, diced
1   tablespoon chili powder
2   teaspoons cumin
1   teaspoon sea salt
2   tablespoons Worcestershire sauce
1   tablespoon Dijon mustard
1   tablespoon maple syrup

Servings: 4   Prep: 20-25 minutes   Cook: 5-6 hours

Soak lentils overnight in water with lemon juice. Drain and rinse before placing into a crock pot. Add the rest of the ingredients to the crockpot with the lentils. Cover and cook in crock pot for 5-6 hours. Lentils should be soft enough to eat.

Serving Suggestions: *Serve with sour cream, open face on a piece of sprouted, whole grain bread, or in a sprouted, whole grain bun. Top with raw cheese.*

Super Sloppies (Sloppy Joe Style)

1	pound grass-fed, organic ground beef
¼	cup onion, chopped
½	cup tomato paste
½	cup organic beef broth
½	tablespoon apple cider vinegar
2	teaspoons cumin
2	teaspoons yellow mustard
1½	teaspoons Worcestershire sauce
½	teaspoon sea salt
2	dashes cayenne
1	dash ground cloves

Servings: 4   Prep: 15 minutes   Cook: 30 minutes

Brown the meat and onions in a large skillet over medium-high heat. Drain meat and put back in skillet. Add the rest of the ingredients and mix well. Simmer 20 minutes and serve.

Serving Suggestions: *Serve with sour cream, open face on a piece of sprouted, whole grain bread, or in a sprouted, whole grain bun. Top with raw cheese. For variation, add ¼ cup chopped celery and/or ¼ cup shredded carrot when meat is almost browned.*

Turkey Taco Salad

1	pound free-range, organic, ground turkey (or ground beef)
2	tablespoons tomato paste
2-3	teaspoons chili powder
1½	teaspoons ground cumin
¼	teaspoon garlic powder
¼	teaspoon onion powder
¼	teaspoon paprika
1	teaspoon sea salt
½	teaspoon black pepper
½	cup organic broth (or water)

Servings: 4   Prep: 10 minutes   Cook: 25 minutes

Brown the turkey in a skillet over medium-high heat. Drain meat and put back in skillet with all of the spices and broth. Simmer about 15 minutes, stirring occasionally.

Serving Suggestions*: Serve over lettuce with shredded raw cheese, tomatoes, black olives, black beans, sour cream or yogurt, and crumbled blue chips (optional). Great with Salsa, page 187 and Guacamole, page 184.*

Vegetable Rice Stir Fry

¼   cup onion, chopped
3   tablespoons coconut oil
3   tablespoons water
2   carrots, chopped
1   red pepper, chopped
½   zucchini, chopped
½   head kale, chopped
3   tablespoons naturally fermented soy sauce
½   teaspoon ground ginger
½   teaspoon garlic or 1 clove, chopped
⅓   cup raw slivered almonds
1   cup brown or wild rice, cooked

Servings: 2-3   *Prep: 25 minutes*   *Cook: 15 minutes*

Sauté the onions in coconut oil over medium-high heat for 3-5 minutes or until tender. Add water and the rest of the vegetables and stir fry in the pan. When vegetables are close to being done add soy sauce, ginger, garlic, and almonds. Stir cooked rice into vegetables and serve.

Serving Suggestions: *Try with quinoa instead of rice.*

Almond Butter-Coconut Crust

⅓   cup raw almond butter
2   tablespoons coconut oil
¼   cup Rapadura* or Sucanat*
½   teaspoon vanilla
1¼   cups brown rice flour*
1   tablespoon dried coconut flakes

Servings: 1 crust   *Prep: 20 minutes*   *Cook: 25 minutes*

Preheat oven to 300°F. In saucepan over low heat, melt almond butter and coconut oil. Remove from heat and stir in Rapadura or Sucanat and vanilla. Slowly add brown rice flour and coconut flakes and mix well. Press into a greased 8 X 8 pyrex dish and refrigerate 15 minutes. Bake at 300°F for 20-25 minutes or until lightly browned.

Serving Suggestions: *Great crust for Apple Bars, page 175 or Cocoa-nut Milk Pudding Bars, page 179.*

Apple Bars

1   Almond Butter-Coconut Crust (page 174)

Apple Topping:
⅓   cup maple sugar or coconut palm sugar*
1   stick organic butter, cold and chopped into 8 pieces
⅔   cup pecans, chopped

Apple Filling:
4-6 apples, peeled, cored, and sliced
¼   cup lemon juice
3   tablespoons maple sugar or coconut palm sugar*
½   teaspoon cinnamon
½   teaspoon vanilla

Servings: 6-8   Prep: 40 minutes   Cook: 60 minutes

Make crust, prebake 10 minutes, and set aside. Preheat oven to 375°F.

To make apple topping: Put the maple or coconut sugar in food processor with butter pieces and pulse until mixture resembles coarse crumbs. Add pecan pieces and pulse a couple more times to combine and set aside.

To make apple filling: Peel, core, and slice the apples and then sprinkle with lemon juice. Mix the rest of the ingredients together and toss with the apples until they are coated. Place into crust and cover with apple topping. Bake at 375°F for 30 minutes covered and then an additional 10 minutes uncovered or until browned and bubbling.

Serving Suggestions: *Serve warm with a side of cream.*

Applesauce Cake

1   cup brown rice or oat flour*
1   teaspoon baking soda
½   teaspoon baking powder
½   teaspoon cinnamon
½   teaspoon cloves
½   cup coconut oil
1   cup coconut palm sugar*
1   free-range, organic egg
1   cup applesauce
½   cup raisins or zante currants* (optional)

Servings: 6   Prep: 15 minutes   Cook: 35 minutes

Preheat oven to 300°F. In a small bowl, mix brown rice or oat flour, baking soda, baking powder, cinnamon, and cloves; set aside. In a large mixing bowl mix coconut oil and coconut palm sugar together until creamy and then add egg and applesauce. Slowly pour the flour mixture into the applesauce mixture and mix completely. Stir the raisins or currants in by hand. Bake in a well greased 8 X 8 inch Pyrex dish (try using coconut oil) at 300°F for approximately 35 minutes.

Serving Suggestions*: Serve with Applesauce.*

Baked Custard

¾   cup organic heavy cream
⅛   teaspoon sea salt
¾   cup coconut milk
2   free-range, organic eggs (beaten)
2   free-range, organic egg yolks (beaten)
3   tablespoons maple sugar or coconut palm sugar*
2   teaspoons vanilla

Servings: 6   Prep: 15 minutes   Cook: 35 minutes

Preheat oven to 350°F. Mix cream with sea salt until slightly thick in food processor (about 2-3 minutes). Add the rest of the ingredients and process until smooth. Pour into 6 small ramekins and place them into a 9 X 13 inch dish, ½ filled with water. Bake for 35 minutes or until firm and lightly browned on top.

Serving Suggestions*: For variation, serve with berries on top.*

Chocolate Brownie Cake

1 ½	cups garbanzo beans (canned or cooked)
¾	cup organic chocolate chips
3	free range, organic eggs
¾	cup coconut palm sugar or sucanat*
¼	cup organic butter (1/2 stick)
1	teaspoon baking powder
¼	teaspoon sea salt
¼	teaspoon vanilla

Servings: 6-8   Prep: 25 minutes   Cook: 3-4 hours

Preheat oven to 350°F. Drain and rinse garbanzo beans and process in a food processor into small pieces. Add remaining ingredients and process again until smooth. Pour into a buttered 8 X 8 inch Pyrex dish. Bake at 350°F for about 30 minutes (use a toothpick to determine that it is cooked). Cool cake and frost, if desired.

Serving Suggestions: *Frost with Chocolate-Fudgy Frosting (below) and/or top with chopped strawberries.*

Chocolate-Fudgy Frosting

2	tablespoons organic heavy cream, yogurt, or almond milk
¼	cup coconut palm sugar or Sucanat*
¼	cup organic chocolate chips
¼	cup raw almond butter or cashew butter
1	tablespoon organic butter

Servings: 1-8X8 cake   Prep: 5 minutes   Cook: 8 minutes

Combine the cream, maple sugar, cocoa, and butter in a heavy saucepan. Stir over medium heat until melted and mixture comes almost to a boil. Add the nut butter and mix well. Let cool for 5 minutes before spreading on cake (has a fudge-like consistency).

Cocoa-nut Milk Pudding

3½ tablespoons raw honey
4½ tablespoons cocoa
⅛   teaspoon powdered stevia*
1½ cups coconut milk
1   pinch sea salt
3   tablespoons arrowroot*
1   tablespoon vanilla

Servings: 6-8   Prep: 15 minutes   Cook: 15 minutes

In pan over low heat, melt honey. Add cocoa and stevia and stir to a chocolate syrup texture. Mix in 3/4 cup of coconut milk and pinch of sea salt. Heat the mixture to just below boiling point. While heating the milk, shake the arrowroot with the remaining 3/4 cup of coconut milk in a small container or jar. Gradually add to the hot milk mixture while stirring. Cook on medium-low heat for approximately 5 minutes or until it begins to thicken, stirring gently. Remove from heat, stir in the vanilla and cool. Refrigerate until thick like a pudding.

Serving Suggestions: Make into Cocoa-nut Milk Pudding Bars (below) or serve cooled with cream on top.

Cocoa-nut Milk Pudding Bars

1   pre-baked, cooled Almond Butter-Coconut Crust (page 174)
1   cooled and refrigerated Cocoa-nut Milk Pudding (see above)
½   cup organic heavy cream, whipped

Servings: 6-8   Prep: 45 minutes   Cook: 35 minutes

Pour cooled pudding into pre-baked pie crust. Top with whipped cream and chill for several hours before serving.

Serving Suggestions: Serve topped with chopped berries.

Nutty Fruit Cobbler

3   cups fresh, or frozen, thawed blueberries (or other fruit)

¼   cup lemon juice

⅔   cup coconut palm sugar or maple sugar*

1½ cups raw pecans or other raw nuts

¾   teaspoon ground cinnamon

1   dash of sea salt

1   stick organic butter, cold and chopped into 8 pieces

Servings: 6   Prep: 10 minutes   Cook: 25 minutes

Preheat oven to 350°F. Place berries in 8 X 8 inch baking dish and sprinkle with lemon juice. In a food processor, combine coconut or maple sugar, pecans, cinnamon, and salt. Add butter pieces to food processor and pulse until mixture resembles coarse crumbs. Sprinkle nut mixture over berries and bake at 350°F for 20-25 minutes or until topping is golden brown and berries are tender.

Serving Suggestions: *Serve warm or cold. A little fresh organic cream is a wonderful accompaniment!*

Vegetable Side Recipes

Coconut Green Beans

1	tablespoon coconut oil
½	cup onion, chopped
2	tablespoons water
2	cloves garlic, minced
1	pound green beans, ends removed
1½	cups tomato, diced
¾	cup coconut milk
½	teaspoon sea salt

Servings: 4-6   *Prep: 10 minutes*   *Cook: 20 minutes*

Sauté onion in coconut oil for 3-5 minutes over medium-high heat. Add water, garlic, and green beans. Stir fry for 8-10 minutes until desired texture. Add tomatoes, coconut milk, and sea salt and heat through.

Serving Suggestions: *Try served over rice or quinoa*.*

Ginger Quinoa Squash

1 butternut squash
½ cup quinoa*
¾ cup water
⅓ teaspoon ginger
1-2 tablespoons organic butter
1 teaspoon raw honey

Servings: 4   Prep: 10 minutes   Cook: 85 minutes

Preheat oven to 300°F. Cut butternut squash in half and remove seeds. Place skin side up into about 1 inch of water in a Pyrex dish and bake at 300°F for about 55 minutes or until tender. While squash is baking, make quinoa by rinsing it and placing it in a saucepan covered with ¾ cup water. Bring water to boil, turn down heat and simmer about 20 minutes or until tender; set aside. Remove cooked squash from skin and mash in a small pan. Stir in ginger and butter and heat over low heat. Add cooked quinoa and top with honey before serving.

Serving Suggestions: *Serve in the skin from the squash.*

Lemon Tahini Kale

1½ tablespoons tahini*
1   tablespoon cold pressed flax oil
1   tablespoon extra virgin olive oil
1   lemon, squeezed
2   teaspoons Ume plum vinegar*
½   teaspoon naturally fermented soy sauce*
1   head kale

Servings: 4   Prep: 10 minutes   Cook: 10 minutes

Combine all ingredients except the kale in a food processor and mix until smooth. Steam kale and chop or tear into pieces. Pour lemon tahini sauce over kale and serve.

Serving Suggestions: *Lemon tahini sauce also makes a great salad dressing!*

Sweet Potato Fries

1   large sweet potato, sliced in strips (peeling optional)
1   tablespoon coconut oil, melted
1   teaspoon sea salt and other spices (optional)
1   tablespoon raw honey* (optional)

Servings: 2-3   Prep: 10 minutes   Cook: 30 minutes

Preheat oven to 300°F. Slice sweet potatoes into strips and put in a large bowl. Cover with coconut oil and stir until coated and sprinkle with sea salt and/or other spices. Spread on cookie sheet and bake at 300°F for about 30 minutes or until soft, turning once. Optional - drizzle some raw honey on top and serve!

Serving Suggestions: *Great snack for children or try with Juicy Hamburgers, page 168.*

Dip and Salsa Recipes

Guacamole Dip

2   avocados
1   lemon, squeezed
1   cup tomato, chopped
¼   cup onion, chopped
2   cloves garlic, minced
2   teaspoons sea salt
¼   teaspoon cayenne

Servings: 4-6   Prep: 10-15 minutes

First scoop avocados out of their shells and mash them in a bowl. Cover with lemon juice to prevent browning. Add remaining ingredients and mix well. Refrigerate 1 hour and serve.

Serving Suggestions: *Great with Turkey Taco Salad, page 172 or Cheese Quesadillas, page 159.*

Hummus Dip

2   cups garbanzo beans (cooked)
2   cloves garlic, crushed
3   tablespoons tahini*
½   cup lemon juice
1   teaspoon cumin
2   dashes cayenne (add to taste)
¼   teaspoon sea salt

Servings: 6   Prep: 15 minutes   Cook: 3-4 hours

Process cooked garbanzo beans in food processor until smooth. Add remaining ingredients and blend to desired consistency. Note: To make smoother, add 2 tablespoons water and 1 tablespoon olive oil.

Serving Suggestions: *Put in bowl and pour 1 tablespoon olive oil over top, sprinkle with paprika, kalamata olives, and parsley.*

Pineapple Chipotle Salsa

2 teaspoons coconut oil
3 cups pineapple, diced
1½ cups onion, chopped
1 cup seeded tomato, diced
2 cloves garlic, minced
½ cup pineapple juice
2 tablespoons coconut palm sugar*
2 tablespoons apple cider vinegar
1 chipotle chile in adobo sauce, drained and minced
1 tablespoon adobo sauce (from drained chiles)
½ cup parsley, finely chopped
2 tablespoons fresh lime juice
½ teaspoon sea salt

Servings: 8   Prep: 10-15 minutes   Cook: 10 minutes

Heat the coconut oil in a large skillet over medium-high heat. Add pineapple and onion, sauté 1 minute or until lightly browned. Add tomato and garlic, sauté 1 minute. Stir in pineapple juice, coconut palm sugar, vinegar, chiles, and adobo sauce. Cook 6 minutes stirring occasionally. Remove from heat and stir in parsley, lime juice, and salt.

Serving Suggestions*: Serve warm over Salmon, page 169, or refrigerate and serve cool as a salsa dip.*

Simply Salsa

1   small Vidalia onion
½   cup cilantro
3   cloves garlic
3   cups tomato, diced
2-4 dashes cayenne (add to desired hotness)
½   lime, squeezed (or use lemon)
¼   teaspoon sea salt

Servings: 8   Prep: 10-15 minutes

In food processor chop onion, cilantro, and garlic. Then add tomatoes and the rest of the ingredients and process until smooth. (Chop and mix by hand for a chunkier salsa.)

Serving Suggestions: *Use jalapeños and use seeds if you want a hotter salsa. Serve with Turkey Taco Salad, page 172 or as salsa dip.*

Zucchini Dip

4   zucchini, shredded (unpeeled)
1   small onion, chopped
1   tablespoon sea salt
Filtered water
1   cup organic, sour cream
2   teaspoons cumin
2   tablespoons lime juice
½   teaspoon fresh ground pepper

Servings: 8   Prep: 15 minutes

Combine zucchini, onion, and sea salt in bowl. Cover with water and soak overnight. Squeeze out in a colander and mix in remaining ingredients. Chill and serve.

Serving Suggestions: *Serve with whole grain crackers.*

Snack Recipes

Almighty Almonds Trail Mix
1   cup raw almonds
½   cup organic raisins
¼   cup dried coconut flakes (optional)

Servings: 3   Prep: 5 minutes

Combine all ingredients and store in airtight container.

Nuts for Chocolate Trail Mix
1   cup raw cashews
1   cup raw pecans
¼   cup organic raisins
¼   cup organic chocolate chips or carob chips

Servings: 3   Prep: 5 minutes

Combine all ingredients and store in airtight container. (Nut mix does not have to include chocolate chips; this is simply a healthier alternative for all of those mixes with the M&M's.)

Pecan Surprise Trail Mix
1   cup raw pecans
1   cup raw pumpkin seeds
1   cup dried cranberries

Servings: 3   Prep: 5 minutes

Combine all ingredients and store in airtight container.

Snack Serving Suggestions*: Try nut mixes using various nuts and dried fruits for fun and healthy snacks!*

Popcorn

¼   cup organic popcorn kernels
2-3 tablespoons coconut oil
3   tablespoons coconut oil and/or butter
1   teaspoon sea salt (add to taste)

Servings: 1-2   Prep: 10 minutes   Cook: 10 minutes

Heat coconut oil in skillet on medium to high heat and add popcorn kernels. (Note: You may want to test just a couple kernels to see if the pan is hot.) Cover and shake pan while corn is popping. Remove from heat. Top the popcorn with melted coconut oil and/or butter and sprinkle with sea salt. Popcorn can also be made in an air popper. This is a popular and fun snack for both children and adults that you can see, hear, smell, and taste!

Serving Suggestions: *For variation in flavor, add things like garlic, nutritional yeast, cayenne pepper, maple syrup, etc.*

Spread Recipes

Cinnamon Coconut Oil Spread
2   tablespoons coconut oil, softened
¼   teaspoon cinnamon
1   teaspoon raw honey*

Servings: 3-4   Prep: 5 minutes

Beat oil, cinnamon, and honey together until smooth. Can be stored covered on the counter or in the refrigerator.

Honey Coconut Butter Spread
2   teaspoons raw honey, melted
1   tablespoon coconut oil, softened
½   stick organic butter, softened

Servings: 4   Prep: 5 minutes

Beat all ingredients together until smooth and creamy. Store covered in the refrigerator.

Strawberry Coconut Butter Spread
2   teaspoons organic strawberry preserves
½   tablespoon coconut oil, softened
½   stick organic butter, softened

Servings: 4   Prep: 5 minutes

Beat all ingredients together until smooth and creamy. Store covered in the refrigerator.

Serving Suggestions for all spreads: *Spread on toast, Cinnamon Waffles, page 153, or French Toast, page 157.*

Section I

Dining Out and Healthy Eating Tips

Dining Out and Healthy Eating Tips

Chew thoroughly, eat slowly and peacefully

Digestion begins with chewing as saliva mixes with food and amylase enzymes begin carbohydrate digestion. Eating slowly allows for proper digestion of food, and gives the brain the opportunity to register fulfillment so you won't overeat. Don't eat while you are preoccupied, stressed, rushing, driving, watching T.V., etc. as this can hinder digestion and lead to uncomfortable consequences. Breathe between bites and enjoy your food!

> **Be Healthy! Tip:** Schedule meals on your calendar or in your day planner like you would any other appointment and sit down at a table in peace.

Eat until you are three-quarters full

Not stuffing yourself leaves room in your stomach for your body to churn food, allowing for better digestion. Slow down when you eat so that your brain can monitor your food intake and let you know when you have had enough. Eating leisurely is a lot more enjoyable than gobbling your food down anyway!

Be Healthy! Tip: Use a smaller dinner plate than you would normally and only take one serving. Wait 30 minutes and see if you really need that second helping of potatoes!

Keep blood sugar stable

Low blood sugar creates an alarm reaction and throws your body into a compensation mode, leading to exhaustion of the glands that maintain your metabolic rate at a high level. It also elevates your levels of insulin, which is your fat storing (weight gaining) hormone. To stabilize your blood sugar, eat at regular intervals and eat protein or fat with each meal or snack.

Be Healthy! Tip: To stabilize your blood sugar, develop the habit of eating every 3 to 4 hours and be sure to include protein and fat with all snacks and meals.

Avoid skipping a meal or excessive calorie reduction

It seems like a good way to lose weight, but, in actuality, skipping meals will push you on the road to obesity! Restriction of calories or starving yourself makes your body think you are starving and your metabolism will actually slow down (which is the opposite of what you want to lose weight). You also disrupt your blood sugar and set yourself up for binges and sweet cravings. Eating actually raises your metabolic rate!

Be Healthy! Tip: Never skip a meal and preferably eat before you get hungry to avoid binging. Carry snacks and lunches with you! Buy a small lunch cooler – visit www.cooltote.com.

Make Healthy Choices When Eating Out

Eating out is something many people enjoy as a social event or sometimes to take a break from cooking and cleaning! There are some choices you can make at a restaurant to ensure that your meal is healthier and is not full of additives, preservatives, and MSG. Choosing finer dining is definitely the way to go as opposed to fast food. Most fast food restaurants use a lot of artificial ingredients. Check around in your local area for restaurants that make their food in-house and have a real chef cooking in the kitchen.

Be Healthy! Tip: Make healthier choices when at a restaurant such as:

- Pass on having the bread basket
- Bring your own sea salt for seasoning
- Bring your own stevia to sweeten your beverage
- Ask for extra vegetables instead of potatoes or pasta
- Ask for grilled foods
- Pass on fried dishes

- Ask for brown or wild rice instead of white rice
- Ask for all sauces and dressings on the side
- Ask for nuts on your salad instead of croutons
- Get sandwiches with romaine instead of a bun
- Pass on desserts other than fruit

Get enzymes in your diet

You are not what you eat, but what you digest and absorb. If you are not eating live, whole, and sometimes raw (preferably organic) foods, then you are probably enzyme deficient. Without adequate enzymes, your body will suffer from indigestion, bloating, gas, constipation, belching, cramping, and/or bad breath. Our natural production of enzymes decreases as we age.

> **Be Healthy! Tip:** Enhance digestion by taking a digestive enzyme. Another idea is to add 1 teaspoon of apple cider vinegar to 2-4 ounces of water and drink with meals.

Maintain healthy gut flora

There are both good and bad forms of bacteria that can proliferate in your gut. It is important to have more good than bad to maintain optimal health. An improper amount of healthy flora has been linked with chronic disease. Eating foods such as kefir to replenish the flora or taking lactobacillus/acidophilus supplements is highly recommended and is especially important if you are taking or have taken an antibiotic for any reason.

> **Be Healthy! Tip:** Enhance gut flora with probiotic supplements or by eating probiotic-rich foods like sauerkraut and kefir. Drink lacto-fermented beverages such as kombucha.

Exercise, specifically rebound exercise

Rebounding is a great way to improve the tone of your digestive system and to stimulate drainage and waste release out of the lymphatic system (and not traumatize the musculoskeletal system). Use of a rebounder has proven to be an efficient form of cardiovascular, body toning, and weight loss enhancing exercise with virtually no harmful side effects. Moreover, it enhances cellular metabolism and energizes every cell with fresh oxygen and nutrients.

> **Be Healthy! Tip:** Buy a rebounder and simply exercise just 5- 10 minutes a day and see the results! Rebounders can add fun to your workout and help you improve balance and circulation, while being easy on your joints. For more information on rebounders or to purchase, visit www.aplacetobe.com.

Drink Water

Drinking water is one of the best ways to maintain optimal health. The human body contains approximately 60% water. Adequate water ingestion is essential for every bodily function. Our bodies use water to help regulate temperature, as well as transport oxygen and nutrients to our cells. Finally, adequate amounts of water can improve digestion, metabolism, and elimination.

> **Be Healthy! Tip:** Take your body weight divided by two and the resultant number is the amount of water you should ingest in ounces. A good investment is a whole house water system to ensure pure water for drinking as well as for showering!

Section II

Organic and Local Buying Tips

Organic and Local Buying Tips

Buying organic products is important not only for the higher quality of food, but also for the impact on our economy and agriculture. As we continue to support the organic and eco-friendly industries, environmental protection and lower pricing on organics will become possible. Whenever possible, try to buy organic or local foods and use the tips in this section to guide you.

The following are ten reasons to buy organic products. Source: Maple Creek Farm in Michigan.

1. Protect Generations

A child can receive four times more exposure to pesticides from food than an adult.

2. Prevent Soil Erosion

Care of the soil is one of the fundamentals of organic farming. In conventional farming, the soil is often just used as a medium for holding plants in a vertical position so that they can be chemically fertilized. North American farms are experiencing the worst soil erosion in history.

3. Protect Water Quality

The Environmental Protection Agency (EPA) estimates that pesticides contaminate the ground water in 38 states, polluting the primary source of drinking water for more than half of the country's population.

4. Save Energy

Modern farming uses more petroleum than any other single industry, consuming 12 percent of the country's total energy supply. More energy is used to produce synthetic fertilizers than to till, cultivate, and harvest crops in North America. Organic farming is more likely to use labor-intensive practices, cover crops, natural fertilizers, and rock powders instead of synthetic fertilizers.

5. Keep Chemicals off Your Plate

Many pesticides approved by the EPA were registered before research had been completed which linked them to cancer and other diseases. Now, the EPA considers many of these substances to be carcinogenic; some are implicated in birth defects, nerve damage, and genetic mutations. The bottom line is that pesticides are poisons designed to kill living organisms and they can also harm humans.

6. Protect Farm Workers

A National Cancer Institute study found that farmers exposed to herbicides had six times more risk of contracting cancer than non-farmers. Field workers suffer high rates of occupational illness.

7. Help Small Farmers

Most organic farms are small, independently-owned family farms. It's estimated that North America has lost more than 650,000 family farms in the past decade. Organic farming could be one of the few survival tactics left for family farms.

8. Support a True Economy

Although organic foods might seem expensive, conventional food prices don't reflect hidden costs, including federal subsidies, pesticide regulation and testing, and hazardous waste disposal and cleanup.

9. Promote Biodiversity

While mono-cropping (growing only one crop year after year) has tripled farm production between 1950 and 1970, the lack of natural diversity of plant life has left the soil lacking natural minerals and nutrients. Single crops are also much more susceptible to pests, making farmers more reliant on pesticides.

Between 1947 and 1974, crop losses due to insects doubled while, at the same time, pesticide use increased.

10. Better Flavor

There's a good reason why many chefs use organic foods in their recipes; they taste better. Foods grown in a nutrient rich soil and picked fresh have a richer flavor (not to mention the freshness, variety, and regional economic benefits of locally produced food).

Where to Buy Organic and Local Foods

Farmers' Markets - Areas where local farmers gather to sell items, normally on a weekly basis. The produce is usually much fresher than you can find at supermarkets and is more likely to be organic. To find a farmers' market in your area, visit www.ams.usda.gov/farmersmarkets/map.htm.

Local Harvest Map - Website allowing you to find all the farmers' markets, family farms, locally-grown produce, grass-fed meats, and other sources of sustainable food in your area. Find the map at www.localharvest.org.

Community Supported Agriculture (CSA) - By joining a CSA, you will gain the benefits of a direct farmer-to-consumer relationship. You then receive fresh produce weekly from the farm you are supporting. This type of commitment will help to sustain local agriculture today and for generations to come. National CSA directory can be found at www.csacenter.org.

Mail Order - There are many companies that ship organic items to consumers nationwide. The foods are expertly packed and shipped, although this is usually a more expensive option. Visit www.diamondorganics.com or www.azurestandard.com.

Local Weston A. Price Foundation Chapter - Supports the research of nutrition pioneer Dr. Weston Price and his studies of optimal diets in our ancestors. The group provides sources for local, organic, and biodynamic vegetables, fruits, grains, and also milk products, butter, eggs, chicken, and meat from pasture-fed animals. Visit www.westonaprice.org for a local chapter near you.

Obtain a Shopping Guide - Weston A. Price Foundation publishes a shopping guide (contact information and brand names listed) for supermarkets and health food stores. Visit www.westonaprice.org to order one.

Organic Pages Online - Provided by the Organic Trade Association (OTA) (www.ota.com) is an easy way to find certified organic products, producers, ingredients, supplies, and services offered by OTA members, as well as items of interest to the entire organic community. Visit www.theorganicpages.com.

Organic Consumers Association - An organization that deals with issues of food safety, industrial agriculture, genetic engineering, corporate accountability, and environmental sustainability. A great resource for finding organic foods, supporting farmers, organics, and the environment. Visit www.organicconsumers.org.

Food Co-ops - Find a food cooperative near you to access reduced pricing in a "buying club" type format with membership. To find out more about a co-op in your area, visit www.unitedbuyingclubs.com.

Health Food Stores - Many health food stores carry local and organic products, fruits, and vegetables. Check around for pricing and availability. Be sure to ask your local stores to carry more organics.

Local Supermarkets - Most supermarkets are now beginning to carry organic and local produce as well as other healthy items. Look for labels such as "locally grown" or "certified organic". Also, ask your grocer to carry more organic and local foods.

Michigan Residents

Obtain a Source Guide - Healthy Traditions Network, the local chapter of the Weston A. Price Foundation, publishes a Michigan Source Guide listing various farmers, including some organic options. Visit www.htnetwork.org.

Obtain an Eating Organically Guide - Michigan Organic Food and Farm Alliance publishes a guide to Michigan's organic and sustainable food producers and related businesses. Visit www.moffa.net.

Obtain a *Taste the Local Difference* Guide - The Michigan Land Use Institute's Entrepreneurial Agriculture Project has a guide to link consumers to farms, grocery stores, restaurants, caterers, and other businesses supporting and featuring local foods. Visit www.localdifference.org.

Join a Local Farm - Maple Creek Farm is a family operation in the thumb area of Michigan which is in their 11th year of growing acres of certified organic produce. They are committed to the growth of CSA and local sustainable organic agriculture. To find a CSA or local farmers near you, visit www.csacenter.org or www.foodroutes.org or www.localharvest.org.

Section III

Cooking and Food Preparation Tips

Cooking and Preparation Tips

Produce Preparation

Washing Tips: Be sure to thoroughly wash produce to get some of the residue off. However, know that you cannot wash all the toxins off if the produce is not organic. For washing both organic and non-organic fruits and vegetables, use Grapefruit Seed Extract (Citricidal) or another vegetable wash found at health food stores.

Cooking Tips: Steam vegetables to retain the most nutrients. You can buy a steamer insert that can fit right into your pan on the stove, or you can use a separate steamer on your counter. Note: When vegetables are boiled, the nutrients end up in the water, which is usually discarded.

Serving Tips: Vegetables are best served with a fat of some sort in order to retain the nutrients that are available in the vegetables. Try serving with butter and unrefined salt to taste. (For sources of unrefined salt, see Chapter 6, "Salt".)

Avoid frying

Do not eat or make any fried foods. Fried foods have been cooked at temperatures so high that it alters the food constituents and creates harmful free radicals. Free radicals are damaging to the cells and tissues of the body.

> **Be Healthy! Tip:**   Try other types of cooking such as baking, steaming, or sautéing.

Avoid microwaves

Microwaving results in reduced or altered minerals, vitamins, and nutrients in food products. Moreover, by-products are often formed in microwaving which are then absorbed, but unable to be broken down in the body. Never microwave food in plastic because it results in leaching of the harmful chemicals and estrogens from the plastic into the food.

> **Be Healthy! Tip:**   Use a toaster oven or convection oven that can heat foods quickly and almost as easily as a microwave.

Avoid aluminum

Aluminum is a highly toxic metal. Large numbers of aluminum molecules enter food that is cooked, covered by, or stored in aluminum pots, pans, cans, and foil. Teflon coatings (also toxic) do not prevent aluminum from leaching into foods. Aluminum toxicity has been linked to memory loss and Alzheimer's disease.

> **Be Healthy! Tip:** Buy stainless steel or cast iron pots and pans to cook with. Use parchment to cover items you are baking instead of foil. Also, you can use parchment paper or unbleached waxed paper to wrap foods for storage.

Avoid plastic

Plastic can contain estrogens and some plastics also have chemicals that can leach into the food and lead to imbalance in the body. It is especially harmful when the plastic is heated and is touching food. Avoid heating items in plastic or covered with plastic. Microwave-safe simply means the item will not crack or melt, but does not mean it will not leach chemicals into your food.

> **Be Healthy! Tip:** Buy Pyrex® glass dishes for reheating. Store items in either the Pyrex® glass dishes or in glass mason jars. Buy a container that is not made of plastic to carry your water, such as a Sigg Bottle at www.sigg.com.

Section IV

Meal Planning and Recipe Conversion Tips

Meal Planning Tips

Food preparation is one of the keys to a healthy diet. It is important to make time for and put energy into what you are going to have for your meals and how you are going to prepare them. Rather than wait until you are stressed out, just getting home from work, or tending to the children, why not plan ahead and save some time and headaches. You can cut down on the time it takes you to grocery shop, as well as how much you spend, by simply planning ahead exactly what you need for your meals and snacks for the week prior to shopping. Use the tips below to assist you in this process.

Ideas for Meal Planning:

Plan meals ahead of time using a meal planner

Using a meal planner such as *The Weekly Meal Planning Tool*™ can help you organize your meals on a weekly basis. There is an area to put in what needs to come out of the freezer beforehand so you don't get to dinnertime and end up with a frozen steak that still needs to be thawed. Also, many people find that planning meals helps to cut down on the urge to just "grab fast food" because you don't know what to make for dinner. Snacks can even be included so you remember to carry them with you each day and can help you avoid those tempting vending machines! You can print *The Weekly Meal Planning Tool*™ for FREE at www.sherylshenefelt.com/shopwithsheryl

Plan weekly meals on Sundays

It makes sense to pick a day to plan your meals. Don't wait until you are just getting home from work. Planning ahead will save time and relieve your stress. Every Sunday, plan the meals you will have for the week, including breakfast, lunch, and dinner. Figure out what ingredients you have and what you may need and then do your grocery shopping for the entire week. See Appendix B for a handy *Grocery Shopping Checklist*. You could even do some of the cooking on Sunday and just use leftovers for meals during the week.

Prepare for meals in the evening

Set aside 15-20 minutes before you go to bed each night to prepare for the following days' meals. You can get out all of the ingredients and also do any of the initial preparation work such as mixing, soaking, chopping or thawing as necessary. The less you have to do after a long day at work, the better!

Get in the habit of carrying a lunch and snacks with you

Use a soft-pack lunch cooler and pack it every night before you go to bed. You can pack leftovers, soups, salads with chicken on top, or other items. And don't forget to always carry nuts, cheese, yogurt, fruits, or vegetables for quick snacks or for times when you are late for a meal. Visit www.cooltote.com for a great lunch pack made with recycled materials.

Get up 15 minutes earlier each day to make breakfast

Take the time to make sure you get a fresh start on the day and prepare breakfast for yourself and/or your family. Don't forget to include some healthy fat for energy to help you through the morning. Conversely, be sure to avoid excess sugar for breakfast. It will start you out with an energy spike, but you more than likely will come crashing down mid-morning. Making a simple smoothie using yogurt, kefir, or coconut milk as a base is an easy and delicious way to start the day!

Schedule meals as an appointment on your calendar

Make meals a priority in your life and in your day. Don't just leave it as an afterthought, as it may never get done. Buy a large calendar for the kitchen to record the planned dates and times of your meals.

Make double or triple batches of any recipes you prepare

Why make a recipe only once? If you double or triple batches, you can have leftovers for meals the next day or to store in the freezer in handy one-serving sizes for the future. Also, try sharing some cooking with a friend and swap portions of the meals you make to add more variety to your eating.

Recipe Conversion Tips

Many of your favorite recipes can be altered to make them healthier. Simply replace some of the ingredients using the ideas below and then test the recipe. Some varying of proportions may be necessary to get the desired results.

Ideas for implementation

- Use natural, whole ingredients for your recipes.
- Avoid canned ingredients.
- Avoid the whites (sugar, flour, salt, pasta).
- Shop for items at a health food store or health aisle of your local grocer to avoid items with unnecessary additives or preservatives.
- Buy items with only the ingredients you would recognize as necessary to make that item.
- Make sure you can pronounce all ingredients on the item you are buying to add to your recipe.
- Use organic items in your recipe, if available.
- Shop from your local farmers' market or from a local farmer whenever possible (resource online at www.localharvest.org).

STEP #1 - Look at fats

- Replace all vegetable or canola oil with butter, ghee, olive oil, or coconut oil.

- Replace margarine or shortening with butter.

NOTE: See charts on Pages 62 and 63 for a summary of how to use various fats and oils as supplements or for cooking.

STEP #2 - Look at flours

- Replace white flour with a whole grain flour – spelt, kamut, and even whole wheat are possible alternatives. Often you will need more whole grain flour than recipe calls for or less liquids. Gluten-free flours such as coconut flour, arrowroot flour, brown rice flour, and nut flours can also be used.

- Explore the use of nuts as well as combinations of grains and nuts.

- Explore soaking of grains for easier digestibility.

NOTE: See recipes involving soaking in Chapter 10. If you are gluten-free, please see the authors' book *The Guide to a Gluten-Free Diet*.

STEP #3 - Look at sweeteners

- Replace white sugar with a natural sweetener. If using a liquid sweetener, then you may need less of the liquid ingredients in the recipe, or more of the flour.

NOTE: To convert white sugar to a natural sweetener, see the chart on Page 43.

STEP #4 - Look at meats

- Use grass-fed, organic, or free-range meats instead of commercial meats laden with antibiotics and hormones. Grass-fed is preferred over grain-fed.
- Buy processed meats that are free of nitrates and nitrites.

NOTE: See resources on Pages 82-83 to find out where to buy quality meats.

STEP #5 - Look at dairy products

- Use whole milk, organic dairy products. Try to find low-heat pasteurized (or raw dairy if accessible).
- Replace condensed milk with real milk or yogurt and a natural sweetener.

- Use plain yogurt and add stevia or fresh fruit instead of buying sweetened yogurts.

- Use yogurt or even kefir instead of milk if you have digestive issues.

NOTE: Visit www.realmilk.com for more information about milk. If you are dairy-free, please see the authors' book **The Guide to a Dairy-Free Diet**. For more about why soy milk is not a good dairy alternative see the authors' book **The Soy Deception**, as well as www.thesoydeception.com.

Appendix A: Glycemic Index of Carbohydrates

The glycemic index is a measure of the speed of entry of carbohydrates into the bloodstream. Since carbohydrates cause blood sugar to rise, resulting in an elevated insulin level, it is recommended to limit the foods with the highest glycemic index and to eat foods with the lowest glycemic index (i.e., those with an index <50%).

High glycemic index, greater than 100% ('Bad' carbohydrates)
Grain-Based Foods
> Puffed rice
> Corn flakes
> Puffed wheat
> Millet
> Instant rice
> Instant potato
> Microwaved potato
> French bread

Simple Sugars
> Maltose
> Glucose

Snacks
> Tofu ice cream
> Puffed-rice cakes

Glycemic Index Standard = 100%
White Bread

Glycemic Index between 80 and 100%

Grain-based foods
    Grape-Nuts
    Whole wheat bread
    Rolled oats
    Oat bran
    Instant mashed potatoes
    White rice
    Brown rice
    Muesli
    Shredded wheat
Vegetables
    Carrots
    Parsnips
    Corn
Fruits
    Banana
    Raisins
    Apricots
    Papaya
    Mango
Snacks
    Ice cream (low fat)
    Corn chips
    Rye crisps

Glycemic index between 50 and 80%

Grain-based foods
    Spaghetti (white)
    Spaghetti (whole wheat)
    Pasta, other
    Pumpernickel bread
Fruits
    Kiwi
    Orange
    Orange juice
Vegetables
    Beets
    Peas
    Sweet potato
    Pinto beans
    Garbanzo beans

Kidney beans (canned)
Baked beans
Navy beans
Simple sugars
Lactose
Sucrose

Glycemic index between 30 and 50%

Grain based foods
Barley
Oatmeal (slow cooking)
Whole grain bread
Fruits
Apple
Apple juice
Applesauce
Grapes
Peaches
Pears
Vegetables
Kidney beans (fresh)
Black-eyed peas
Chick-peas
Lima beans
Tomato soup
Dairy Products
Ice cream (high fat)
Milk
Yogurt

Glycemic index less than 30% ('Good' carbohydrates)

Fruits
Cherries
Plums
Grapefruit
Vegetables
Green vegetables
Lentils
Simple sugars
Fructose
Nuts

Appendix B: Grocery Shopping Checklist

Print a FREE *Shopping Checklist* you can carry with you to the store at www.sherylshenefelt.com/shopwithsheryl

Fruit, Fresh	Vegetables, Fresh	Vegetables, Frozen
O Avocados	O Arugula	O Asparagus
O Apples	O Asparagus	O Broccoli
O Applesauce	O Basil	O Corn
O Apricots	O Bell Peppers (type'?)	O Green beans
O Bananas		O Lima beans
O Blueberries	O Broccoli	O Peas
O Blackberries	O Carrots (type?)	O Potatoes
O Cantaloupes		O Mixed veggies
O Grapes, Red	O Celery	O
O Grapes, Green	O Cilantro	O
O Honeydew	O Cucumber	O
O Lemons	O Garlic	O
O Limes	O Green beans	
O Nectarines	O Kale	
O Oranges	O Lettuce (type?)	
O Peaches		
O Pineapples	O Onions (type?)	**Fruit, Frozen**
O Raspberries		O Blueberries
O Strawberries	O Potatoes (type?)	O Blackberries
O Watermelons		O Mangoes
O	O Spinach	O Peaches
O	O Sprouts	O Raspberries
O	O Swiss Chard	O Strawberries
O	O Tomatoes	O Tropical blend
	O Squash	O
	O	O
	O	

Fats/Oils
- O Butter
- O Coconut oil
- O Coconut milk
- O Flax oil
- O Ghee
- O Olive oil
- O Palm oil
- O
- O

Canned Goods
- O Artichoke hearts
- O Beans (black, chili, white, garbanzo)
- O Fruits (pineapple, papaya)
- O Olives (black, green)
- O Pizza sauce
- O Sockeye salmon
- O Spaghetti sauce
- O Tomatoes (whole, diced, crushed)
- O Tomato sauce
- O Tomato paste
- O Tuna fish
- O Chicken broth
- O Beef broth
- O
- O

Nut/Seed Butters
- O Almond butter
- O Cashew butter
- O Macadamia nut butter
- O Peanut butter
- O Tahini (sesame seed butter)
- O
- O

Baking
- O Baking powder
- O Baking soda
- O Chocolate chips
- O Cocoa
- O Flours (type?)
- O Honey, raw
- O Maple syrup
- O Spices (type?)
- O Stevia
- O Sweeteners
- O Vanilla
- O
- O

Pasta and Rice
- O Elbow pasta
- O Soba noodles
- O Spaghetti noodles
- O Lasagna noodles
- O Brown rice
- O Wild rice
- O
- O

Breads/Grains
- O Bagels, sprouted
- O Bread, gluten-free
- O Bread, sprouted
- O Buns, sprouted
- O Buckwheat cereal
- O Oats
- O Tortillas, gluten-free
- O Tortillas, sprouted
- O
- O

Nuts and Seeds
- O Almonds
- O Cashews
- O Macadamia nuts
- O Pecans
- O Pine nuts
- O Pumpkins seeds
- O Sesame seeds
- O Sunflower seeds
- O Walnuts
- O
- O

Snacks
- ○ Applesauce
- ○ Blue tortilla chips
- ○ Chips (type?)
- ○ Crackers (type?)
- ○ Dried fruit (apples, apricots, cranberries, raisins)
- ○ Fruit leather
- ○
- ○

Meats
- ○ Bacon
- ○ Chicken sausages
- ○ Hot dogs
- ○ Meatballs
- ○ Pepperoni
- ○ Sliced meats (turkey, ham, chicken)
- ○ Turkey sausages
- ○
- ○

Dairy and Eggs
- ○ Butter
- ○ Cheese (mild, sharp, Colby, Monterey Jack)
- ○ Cheese, goat
- ○ Cream
- ○ Cream cheese
- ○ Eggs
- ○ Milk
- ○ Mozzarella
- ○ Parmesan cheese
- ○ Yogurt, plain
- ○
- ○

Beverages
- ○ Amazake
- ○ Beer, microbrew
- ○ Coconut water
- ○ Kombucha
- ○ Wine, sulfite free
- ○ Sake
- ○ Sparkling water
- ○
- ○

Condiments
- ○ Apple cider vinegar
- ○ Balsamic vinegar
- ○ Ketchup
- ○ Kimchi
- ○ Lemon juice
- ○ Lime juice
- ○ Mayo
- ○ Mustard
- ○ Pickles
- ○ Salsa
- ○ Sauerkraut
- ○ Tamari
- ○
- ○

Desserts
- ○ Chocolate
- ○ Ice cream
- ○ Macaroons
- ○ Shortbread
- ○
- ○

About the Authors

David Brownstein, M.D.

David Brownstein, M.D. is a family physician who utilizes the best of conventional and alternative therapies. He is the Medical Director for the Center for Holistic Medicine in West Bloomfield, MI. He is a graduate of the University of Michigan and Wayne State University School of Medicine. Dr. Brownstein is board certified by the American Academy of Family Physicians. He is a member of the American Academy of Family Physicians and the American College for the Advancement in Medicine. He is the father of two beautiful girls, Hailey and Jessica, and is a retired soccer coach.

Dr. Brownstein has lectured internationally about his success with using natural items. Dr. Brownstein has authored *Salt Your Way to Health, 2nd Edition*; *Iodine, Why You Need It, Why You Can't Live Without It, 5th Edition*; *The Miracle of Natural Hormones 3rd Edition*; *Overcoming Thyroid Disorders, 2nd Edition*; *Overcoming Arthritis*; *Drugs That Don't Work and Natural Therapies That Do, 2nd Edition*; *The Guide to Healthy Eating, 2nd Edition*; *The Guide to a Gluten-Free Diet, 2nd Edition*; *The Guide to a Dairy-Free Diet*; and *The Soy Deception*.

Dr. Brownstein is the author of *Dr. Brownstein's Natural Way to Health* Monthly Newsletter. His weekly blog can be accessed on his website at www.drbrownstein.com.

Dr. Brownstein's office is located at:
Center for Holistic Medicine
5821 W. Maple Rd., Ste. 192
West Bloomfield, MI 48323

P: 248.851.1600

www.centerforholisticmedicine.com
www.drbrownstein.com

Follow Dr. B on Facebook at:
www.facebook.com/drdavidbrownstein

Sheryl Shenefelt, C.N., CMTA

Sheryl Shenefelt is a Certified Nutritionist, Certified Metabolic Typing® Advisor, and co-author of *The Guide to Healthy Eating, 2nd Edition; The Guide to a Gluten-Free Diet, 2nd Edition; The Guide to a Dairy-Free Diet;* and *The Soy Deception* with Dr. Brownstein.

As a nutritional consultant and holistic health coach, Sheryl is dedicated to serving the nutritional, lifestyle and wellness needs of individuals and families. As an author, educator, and mother with a passion for studying and researching food and nutrition information, Sheryl works directly with clients, but also teaches workshops aimed at improving the nutritional status and overall health of participants such as her "Shop with Sheryl" classes. She is a past board member of Healthy Traditions Network, the Local Chapter of the Weston A. Price Foundation and is now serving on their advisory board. Sheryl is married to her wonderful husband Bob and has two beautiful children Grace (twelve-years-old) and Nick (eight-years-old); the inspiration for her interest in health and nutrition, and her desire to eat properly and raise a healthy family. "From my experience as a nutritionist and as a wife and mother desiring a healthy family," Sheryl says. "I recognize the importance of carefully selecting the type of food we eat, knowing where our food comes from, and buying foods in their most natural state from local farmers whenever possible."

For more about Sheryl and to join her blog and community and get her recommended products as well as resources for organic, natural, and gluten-free items visit her website at www.sherylshenefelt.com.

Follow Sheryl on Facebook at:
www.facebook.com/aplacetobe

Books by David Brownstein, M.D.

More information: www.drbrownstein.com

Vitamin B12 for Health

Vitamin B12 deficiency is occurring in epidemic numbers. This book show you the many benefits of using natural, bioidentical forms of vitamin B12 and how B12 supplements can help you achieve your optimal health. B12 therapy can treat many common ailments including:

- Anemia
- Autoimmune Illness
- Blood Clots
- Brain Fog
- Cognitive Decline

- Depression
- Fatigue
- Fibromyalgia
- Heart Disease
- Muscle Disease

- Neurologic Problems
- Osteoporosis
- AND MUCH MORE!

IODINE: WHY YOU NEED IT, WHY YOU CAN'T LIVE WITHOUT IT, 5th EDITION

Iodine is the most misunderstood nutrient. Dr. Brownstein shows you the benefit of supplementing with iodine. Iodine deficiency is rampant. It is a world-wide problem and is at near epidemic levels in the United States. Most people wrongly assume that you get enough iodine from iodized salt. Dr. Brownstein convincingly shows you why it is vitally important to get your iodine levels measured. He shows you how iodine deficiency is related to:

- Breast cancer
- Hypothyroidism and Graves' disease
- Autoimmune illnesses
- Chronic Fatigue and Fibromyalgia
- Cancer of the prostate, ovaries, and much more!

OVERCOMING ARTHRITIS

Dr. Brownstein shows you how a holistic approach can help you overcome arthritis, fibromyalgia, chronic fatigue syndrome, and other conditions. This approach encompasses the use of:

- Allergy elimination
- Detoxification
- Diet
- Natural, bioidentical hormones
- Vitamins and minerals
- Water

DRUGS THAT DON'T WORK and
NATURAL THERAPIES THAT DO, 2nd Edition

Dr. Brownstein's newest book will show you why the most commonly prescribed drugs may not be your best choice. Dr. Brownstein shows why drugs have so many adverse effects. The following conditions are covered in this book: high cholesterol levels, depression, GERD and reflux esophagitis, osteoporosis, inflammation, and hormone imbalances. He also gives examples of natural substances that can help the body heal.

See why the following drugs need to be avoided:

- Cholesterol-lowering drugs (statins such as Lipitor, Zocor, Mevacor, and Crestor and Zetia)
- Antidepressant drugs (SSRI's such as Prozac, Zoloft, Celexa, Paxil)
- Antacid drugs (H-2 blockers and PPI's such as Nexium, Prilosec, and Zantac)
- Osteoporosis drugs (Bisphosphonates such as Fosomax and Actonel, Zometa, and Boniva)
- Diabetes drugs (Metformin, Avandia, Glucotrol, etc.)
- Anti-inflammatory drugs (Celebrex, Vioxx, Motrin, Naprosyn, etc)
- Synthetic Hormones (Provera and Estrogen)

SALT YOUR WAY TO HEALTH , 2nd Edition

Dr. Brownstein dispels many of the myths of salt—salt is bad for you, salt causes hypertension. These are just a few of the myths Dr. Brownstein tackles in this book. He shows you how the right kind of salt--unrefined salt--can have a remarkable health benefit to the body. Refined salt is a toxic, devitalized substance for the body. Unrefined salt is a necessary ingredient for achieving your optimal health. See how adding unrefined salt to your diet can help you:

- Maintain a normal blood pressure
- Balance your hormones
- Optimize your immune system
- Lower your risk for heart disease
- Overcome chronic illness

THE MIRACLE OF NATURAL HORMONES, 3RD EDITION

Optimal health cannot be achieved with an imbalanced hormonal system. Dr. Brownstein's research on bioidentical hormones provides the reader with a plethora of information on the benefits of balancing the hormonal system with bioidentical, natural hormones. This book is in its third edition. This book gives actual case studies of the benefits of natural hormones.

See how balancing the hormonal system can help:

- Arthritis and autoimmune disorders
- Chronic fatigue syndrome and fibromyalgia
- Heart disease
- Hypothyroidism
- Menopausal symptoms
- And much more!

OVERCOMING THYROID DISORDERS, 2nd Edition

This book provides new insight into why thyroid disorders are frequently undiagnosed and how best to treat them. The holistic treatment plan outlined in this book will show you how safe and natural remedies can help improve your thyroid function and help you achieve your optimal health. NEW SECOND EDITION!

- Detoxification
- Diet
- Graves'
- Hashimoto's Disease
- Hypothyroidism
- And Much More!!

THE GUIDE TO HEALTHY EATING, 2nd Edition

Which food do you buy? Where to shop? How do you prepare food? This book will answer all of these questions and much more. Dr. Brownstein co-wrote this book with his nutritionist, Sheryl Shenefelt, C.N. Eating the healthiest way is the most important thing you can do. This book contains recipes and information on how best to feed your family. See how eating a healthier diet can help you:

- Avoid chronic illness
- Enhance your immune system
- Improve your family's nutrition

THE GUIDE TO A GLUTEN-FREE DIET, 2nd Edition

What would you say if 16% of the population (1/6) had a serious, life-threatening illness that was being diagnosed correctly only 3% of the time? Gluten-sensitivity is the most frequently missed diagnosis in the U.S. This book will show how you can incorporate a healthier lifestyle by becoming gluten-free.

- Why you should become gluten-free
- What illnesses are associated with gluten sensitivity
- How to shop and cook gluten-free
- Where to find gluten-free resources

THE GUIDE TO A DAIRY-FREE DIET

This book will show you why dairy is not a healthy food. Dr. Brownstein and Sheryl Shenefelt, CCN, will provide you the information you need to become dairy free. This book will dispel the myth that dairy from pasteurized milk is a healthy food choice. In fact, it is a devitalized food source which needs to be avoided.

Read this book to see why common dairy foods including milk cause:

- Osteoporosis
- Diabetes
- Allergies
- Asthma
- A Poor Immune System

THE SOY DECEPTION

This book will dispel the myth that soy is a healthy food. Soy ingestion can cause a myriad of severe health issues. More information can be found online at: www.thesoydeception.com. Read this book to see why soy can cause:

- Allergies
- Cancer
- Osteoporosis
- Thyroid Disorders
- A Poor Immune System
- And, Much More!